THE INFINITY DIET:
GUIDE TO WEIGHT LOSS
& LONGEVITY

MICHAEL SCHLIE

The Infinity Diet: Guide to Weight Loss & Longevity

Copyright © 2017 by Michael J. Schlie

First Edition
First Revision

ISBN-13: 978-1544633060
ISBN-10: 1544633068

www.theinfinitydiet.com

Table of Contents

Preface vii

Chapter 1 What Does Science Say? 1

Chapter 2 Are You Willing To Change? 7

Chapter 3 Can I Do This? 13

Chapter 4 How Did We Get Here? 19

Chapter 5 I Thought This Was A Diet Book!!! 31

Chapter 6 How Do I Start? 47

Chapter 7 I Can Eat What!!!! 53

Chapter 8 What Does Exercise Have To Do With Diet? ... 65

Chapter 9 What Is This Alkaline Stuff All About? 73

Chapter 10 This Diet Doesn't Have Pills? 79

Chapter 11 So You Need To Learn How To Cook 83

Chapter 12 You Mean I Can Cheat!!! 93

Chapter 13 The Outside Factor 99

Chapter 14 Is Your Peach Really A Peach? 109

Chapter 15 You Should Know Chapter 115

Conclusion 139

Index 141

About The Author 151

Dedication

This book is dedicated to everyone who is currently facing extreme medical issues. If one person's health is impacted by these writings, the book will be a tremendous success. For those who want to prevent future health problems, you deserve credit as well. Please spread the gospel of health and use this book as a tool to keep our human race away from the ultimate corporate destruction. To the individuals who deserve some love and recognition for the creation of this book. I give great thanks. First is to my daughter Sam. Thank you, baby, for being my inspiration. Without you, this book would have been just a pipe dream. To both my friends Al. Thank you for keeping my head in the right direction and offering some great stories to feed my message. To my mom, Sheila, I hope you use some of these tools in this book and thank you for having me. You get the ultimate credit. To Selina, thank you for that wonderful talk which sent me on my path to health. I may not be here without you once caring about me.

Preface

OUR SOCIETY IS CHANGING at an alarming rate and the issues we face today are unique. Since the beginning of civilization, humankind has never faced the problems we have created for ourselves. The industrial revolution has changed our environment and our health tremendously since the first machines picked cotton and made blankets. This revolution has caused an evolution, of sorts. What it created was an unhealthy evolution for the earth and all of its creatures. The blame for this catastrophe is the person you see in the mirror, your neighbor and every human in any industrialized nation for the past 300 years. Some people deserve more of the blame than others, but we are all guilty. Overall, every one of us has and will continue to harm the only planet we will ever know, myself included.

The largest common ingredient is wealth and the desire to acquire as much as possible. The quest for greed has caused the destruction of our health and environment. It's an epidemic. The sacrifice this planet and its creatures have endured is incredible, due to this superficial entity called money. It is beyond explanation what people will do for their personal pursuit of this destructive necessity in today's society.

To have true wealth, you must have health. A sick rich person could be miserable while a poor healthy person might have better means to enjoy life. Money creates an illusion of having everything while our health takes a back seat. Can we change as a society and save what humanity hasn't already destroyed? This author isn't quite sure, but I know if each individual did their part, a difference can be achieved. This change needs to start with a few CEO's realizing that rich people won't need their money if everyone else is dead. Someone at the top has to start this trend and it has to begin through the media.

The media and all its advertisers control our brains. For instance, if a movie star said that drinking goat urine was good for us and it was fortified with vitamin A, C, and protein, goat urine would become very popular. People are mostly ignorant and are followers by nature. The company pushing this product would have a strong influence on other industries, such as the bottling company who has ties with plastics industry who also would have ties with Big Oil and so on. All these companies would want more goat urine to be sold for the name of profit. Why do people buy these types of products anyway? The smoke and mirrors effect is what makes these products more attractive. Look mom, this goat urine has vitamins!!! Please mom, will you buy it for me? What I see is a product of little value, being fortified with a bunch of false hope to create maximum profits. Doesn't this sound like today's breakfast cereal or what? How do we change this mentality? To change human nature is nearly impossible. People tend to see only the good in this world of illusion. Marketing people have this knowledge and they pray on our tendencies.

Now, what can be done about our environment? Does anyone care about the trash island in the middle of the Pacific Ocean the size of Texas? We should since we created this problem and it needs to be cleaned up now. When will we stop using fossil fuel? The technology has been in existence before the first car was invented, however, there were fewer profits in electric cars compared to gas cars. So for the sake of profits, our bones now contain between 1000 and 3000% of the normal levels of heavy metals such as lead and mercury in only 200 years. Has anyone ever heard of autism and fibromyalgia? The CEO's have to realize their children and grandchildren are just as unhealthy as the children living in the projects in Compton. These pollutants affect everyone. Big changes have to be made.

When it comes to death, this author believes when it's our time to go, it should be our decision to die. We can kill ourselves through our lack of desire to live in as little as two weeks. This is why I am so against greed dictating our life expectancy. When Big Business creates bad health for the sake of profits, this is unacceptable. Man made illnesses are created by tainting our food supply through poor dietary options. The ignorant become the prey of Big Medical and Big Pharma caused by Big Food. So where is Johnny? Sick and poor. Where's his health and wealth? Big Business took it from him. When his health and wealth run out, Big Insurance leaves Johnny with the little guy, the undertaker. Johnny has lost it all. Even after he's gone, Big Government gets what's left through death taxes.

This book is a guide to longevity. The Infinity Diet is based on years of research on the requirements of the body and how to maintain a high quality of life until death. This book can bring you both health and wealth. Health to your body and wealth of knowledge. I want humans to survive. This is the main reason I wrote this book. I have a daughter and I hope to have normal grandchildren. It is my desire to have my grandchildren live healthy lives along with everyone else on this planet. Future generations deserve to live like our great grandparents did without all the environmental damage to our Earth and all its inhabitants.

The premise of my research was to see what the body needs without the use of the mind. Our minds play a huge role in controlling our well-being. By eliminating the decision making aspect of health, the body can't be tempted or swayed in any indifferent direction. This program is solely based on what science says about our body's nutritional needs and how to survive until the will to die takes over. This book outlines the very best longevity tools I could find. Many clinical trials and studies were reviewed to determine the optimal nutritional benefits based on results of all the various elements of optimal health. This diet isn't a diet as much as a lifestyle change.

This book wasn't written by a doctor. This book was written by an engineer. I decided to tackle the human body as an engineering project. At first, I started to learn how the human body really works, instead of the untruths we are commonly told. There is a huge difference. Since I wasn't limited by courses taught by pharmaceutical controlled professors and universities, I was able to branch out to discover the true inner workings of the human body. The next step was to figure out what is the body's chemical relationship to the nutrients we eat, breathe and drink. This interaction between function and nutrients brought me to write this book. The information I have uncovered is essential to experiencing a high quality of life for many years after our normal life expectancy. Only a few books I have ever read changed my life. I hope this book changes yours.

Shall we begin?

CHAPTER 1:
What Does Science Say?

SO WHAT DOES SCIENCE SAY? Actually, science says a lot. Science tells us that we're not doing a very good job. We have to become more conscious about our health and as a society; our grade is a D-. This grade needs to improve drastically. The worst part is our health affects our children's health. The food we eat is the same food our children eat, especially in the womb and while breastfeeding. The hardest part to accept is that our great grandparent's health affected our own well-being.

For example, maybe our great grandparents migrated across the ocean and had to breathe the exhaust fumes from the boat coming to Ellis Island. Those fumes were full of toxins that entered their bodies. The water they were drinking back then was pretty pure, except for a little fossil fuel pollution, like lead and mercury. When our grandparents had their children, each baby took in more toxins than the previous one, because of accumulated pollution in the air and water. This was caused by the rapid growth of the Industrial Revolution. Maybe grandpa went to work in the coal mines. Grandpa was no doubt contaminated with pollutants and heavy metals in the workplace. Anyway, all his kids were pretty normal and lived healthy lives. Now his children were old enough to have their own children. The pollutants our great grandparents accumulated were passed on to their children and on to their grandchildren. The next generation seemed normal except for the last child. He had a hard time communicating and was an introvert. Maybe he didn't like crowds and had few friends. His behaviors were the first visible sign of generational toxic poisoning.

Today, 20% of the children have some type of issue. Either ADHD, autism, violent tendencies or even cancer. When will every child born have issues? Common sense should tell us that we need to change our ways as a society. Not tomorrow, but now. Most of our minds are so clouded by these polluting agents taking over our bodies, many of us don't even notice the difference. The lack of quality food choices adds to this fog because the food is lacking the elements needed to think clearly, such as oxygen and good fats. By making small dietary changes and detoxifying the harmful compounds that lay within our bones and cells, we can begin to work on the most important facets of health.

Our body's foundation includes 3 key components. Since this book is about the physical body, we will only explore the physical elements. These components are internal function, endoskeletal system, and endoskeletal muscular system. All three are integral in keeping our bodies healthy into our senior years. If any of these elements are not working correctly, our quality of life will suffer or fail. If we experience failure in any of these key areas, severe issues such as death or a reduction in the quality of life may occur. If we nourish these components correctly through proper diet and exercise, our bodies will flourish and the quality of life will increase. So if we know that taking care of our bodies is so important, why do so many of us disregard our own wellbeing? I believe it is due to laziness or inconvenience. Humans want the easiest possible solution. It's the "give me a pill or "do it for me" type of mentality that holds many of us back. I'm starting to see an evolution in today's people. An awakening, of sorts. People are starting to see many of these issues with their own eyes and it's beginning to drive them to better themselves. We can't depend on doctors anymore to maintain our health. The average doctor has about 7 minutes to diagnose their patients today and our overall trust in doctors is lacking. People are starting to realize that their health depends on themselves and no one else.

Most people I interview are so fed up with the medical industry because their prescribed treatments seem to make them sicker. This is a scary world for the ill. How does society change this broken system? It is only broken for the patients, not medical industry. It is working wonderfully for doctors and insurance companies because of record profits. So what can we do? I suggest looking at what science says regarding our health and make some changes on our own. Life is meant to be enjoyed by being healthy. Health starts with our lungs, stomach and skin and illness starts with our lungs, stomach, and skin. Our body depends on us to choose the right foods, breathe quality air and drink healthy liquids. It is our responsibility to take care of our needs and no one else, except maybe our children. The medical industry doesn't care about our health, only their wealth, so wake up and make the changes yourself. The most critical of all these elements is our internal function.

The internal function is all of the critical parts of our body needed to live, such as organs and glands. We might be able to live without a certain part of our body, but it's much better if all the components are healthy. I believe bad habits and ignorance play a huge role in our health. The lack of desire to better ourselves causes some of these issues. Many people today lack a sense of urgency. It's the "I will take care of it later" mentality dictating our lack of desire for betterment. It is only when a health scare or a lack of social recognition occurs that triggers this sense of urgency. Unfortunately, our body's organs and glands usually receive the most damage from our bad behaviors.

For some people, a lack of knowledge leads to a false sense of well-being. I have heard so many people believe that our food, air, and water are perfectly fine. Why would anyone put toxic materials in our necessities to hurt us? The power of greed has taken precedence over health. Who suffers the most? All of humanity suffers from this quest for wealth. Our food, air, and water should be natural. Anything man made should be regarded as unhealthy. Look at the ingredients in most health care products. What do you see? I see a bunch of chemicals. Did nature put those chemicals in their products? I don't think so. What science says is to eat natural living foods giving to this Earth. These foods will support your internal function and keep you nourished and healthy.

The Endo-skeletal System is our bones, tendons, cartilage, and ligaments. In order to keep this system healthy, we need to watch our food, air, and water intake. Many of these components start to lose their ability to support other body parts as they deteriorate with age. These conditions can be prevented by understanding how the body works through proper nutrients and exercise. This is the intent of this book. For instance, osteoporosis can be prevented, halted or improved by making dietary changes and exercise to support our Endo-skeletal function. Everything needs work in balance. Unfortunately, few people live their lives in balance. If your body is not working correctly, change what you're doing. I once asked a doctor "it hurts when I do this", he said, "Stop doing that". It makes a lot of sense. This pertains to everything we do. If we know that football can lead to Post Concussion Syndrome which causes severe depression and mental issues, so why do we play football? Think about it.

Most people believe they are indestructible until they destruct. It always takes a wake-up call to make people realize that they're damaging their bodies. The difference between the internal function and the Endoskeleton system is that internal function is rarely seen because it is beneath our skin and the Endo-skeletal System is visible. We become more critical of our Endo-skeletal System because we can see the damage and so can others. Unless we caused severe damage to this system earlier in our life, most of the damage can be reversed through diet and exercise. The exercise is to strengthen the ligaments and tendons which allow us to regain some of the flexibility we lost as children.

The Endoskeleton Muscular System is what feeds our bones with nutrients. If this system is neglected, our bones will begin to fail and become brittle. The best way to support this system is to work the muscle surrounding each bone and to eat a proper diet. One of the best treatments for bone health is balance exercises, such as yoga. When your body has to balance, every muscle is engaged to prevent you from falling.

As we age, our ability to balance is lost by the lack of use. As children, we used to walk on curbs and railroad tracks. These movements engaged our whole muscular system. Today, most people live sedimentary lifestyles. To feed your bones and muscles, find time to re-engage these types of activities. By doing so, you will regain these lost abilities.

Diet also plays a huge role in muscle health. Our muscle's main food source is protein. Protein is needed to maintain and repair the damage we incur on a daily basis. Most repairs are done during our sleeping hours. If we don't eat enough protein, our muscles will shrink and will become malnourished. If we eat too much protein, we can experience kidney issues and bone loss.

The muscular system is the main component of The Infinity Diet to maintain our metabolism. Muscle requires an incredible amount of calories, actually 50 calories per pound, for maintenance. If we continually work on our muscle, we can combat the muscle loss associated with the aging process and reduce our body fat content. Studies have shown that by increasing your muscle mass as we age, the aging process is either halted or reversed if we adhere to a healthy diet.

An overview of The Infinity Diet is to eat live healthy foods and to increase our muscle mass throughout our lives. If followed, we will age very slowly and remain healthy until we choose not to live anymore. Our lifestyle, good or bad, can dictate how long we live and at what quality. How valuable is it for you to live without illness and achieve a much longer life span? You can only answer this question. Some people may give this book to the Goodwill after they read it and others may buy additional copies and give them out to their friends. I personally want my friends to live long, healthy lives. No one wants to be lonely, right? This book is only a tool. You can use this book as fuel to self-enrichment or it can be used as a fuel in the fireplace. It is your choice what you want to do with this information.

CHAPTER 2:

Are You Willing To Change?

SOME PEOPLE ARE RESISTANT to change because of comfortability. Many of us won't stray too far from these boundaries. Other people love the excitement of a new adventure and welcome changes in their lives. As we age, we tend to stick to what we already know. This is unfortunate. Changing is a willingness to adapt and progress as a person. If we refuse to change, we fall into the same patterns and eventually become stagnant. This complacency will gradually lead to increasing the likelihood of having health issues, either mentally or physically. By keeping an open mind, your willingness to improve will allow your body to expand its horizons. Are you a go-getter or are you complacent? Look in the mirror. Who knows yourself better than you?

People also tend to be more critical of others and less critical of themselves. It's easy to see flaws in others, but it takes a lot of work to see your own deficiencies. To see yourself, you first have to look into your past. This is very frightening to many. If you have endured traumatic experiences, change may be difficult because of your comfort zone. Take change a little slower, since this isn't a race. It's a lifestyle adjustment. What you want to achieve is a higher quality of life with little physical limitations. Since there isn't a time limit, you can determine the finish line. Isn't this the way life should be? Open yourself up to see the bigger picture.

Since most of our personalities are forged before our 6th birthday, we have little choice but to be the person we are. If traumatic experiences had occurred, these events can alter who we are. We probably all know someone, if not ourselves, who became a different person after a horrible event. However, to change willingly is an accomplishment, for good or for the worse. Realization is the first step to self-improvement. Our human nature resists this action and it takes considerable inner strength to welcome such an event through the use of our willpower.

It seems heredity also plays a part in our reluctance to change. Some families have had the same business and habits for generations and their lifestyle is so embedded in every facet of their lives. Anything out of the ordinary can cause panic like symptoms. In order for these people to open up to new ideas, it takes a tremendous amount of energy. This energy has to come from deep within if they want to improve their quality of life.

Tragedy, social recognition and health scares are the 3 main reasons why people make life changing decisions when it pertains to their health. Everyone has lost a loved one too early from some unforeseen illness. This person probably didn't take care of themselves and they put their health on the back burner. When this person either passed away or never fully recovered, this event can spark our desire to survive. We may see similarities between ourselves and that person so we may start the process of changing your life. This happened in Baseball. When Tony Gwynn died at 54 from salivary gland cancer, many ballplayers stopped using chewing tobacco. Everyone knows it is bad for us, but it doesn't hit home until a tragedy occurs.

We also know people who won't change even through tragedy. My mother is one of these people. I lost my grandfather to Congestive Heart Failure when he was 70. He smoked about 3 packs of cigarettes a day for his whole life. My grandfather used to take himself off his oxygen to smoke. He continued to smoke until the day he died. He vowed he would die with a cigarette in his hand. He almost did. When he passed, he was 5'10" and 85 lbs. My mother witnessed his decline and vowed to herself to never be like him. 20 years later, my mother (who also smokes 3 packs a day) is experiencing the same fate as her grandfather. She vowed she would die with a cigarette in her mouth. Instead of reversing this condition, she has chosen to let it continue. I recently asked her if her father's death meant anything to her.

She said that she didn't want to die in the same manner. She has chosen the same path and is unwilling to put in the effort to save herself from the same self-inflicted illness. So tragedy only works if it touches us deeply enough. Social recognition, peer pressure and mean individuals can trigger a willingness to change in some people. Instead of having the ability to progress on their own, it takes another person's words to activate the change mechanism in our brain. Maybe it's a boyfriend who says your butt is too big or a circle of friends who are extremely thin. Another person being critical of your appearance can activate the "I'll show you" mechanism. These triggers can motivate a person to change. As unhealthy of a decision as it may be, the desire to act should be complimented. Whatever helps you to find that drive is the main goal of making change a reality.

This type of motivation can create an unhealthy behavioral issue called obsession. This condition almost killed a gym owner's client. He and I had to do an intervention several times to curb this person's destructive behavior. Her boyfriend kept making derogatory comments about her appearance. Her obsession to overcome his perceptions almost became fatal. She was fainting and overtraining. She would go days without food. It became a very serious health issue. Through tough love and understanding, she finally changed her habits and returned to her previously happy self. The biggest change for her was dropping that boyfriend. It appears there is a fine balance between change and obsession. Change is a healthy, while obsession is a destructive behavior.

For myself, a few of life-altering events have changed my outlook over the years. Ever since I was about 5 years old, I had kidney problems, however nothing too extensive until I was 31. I lived a partying lifestyle and I felt indestructible like many young adults do. All of a sudden, I started to feel strange, not like myself and very low on energy. I started to have a strong body odor and had eruptions all over my body. My urine became a dark/brownish yellow color and it smelled horrible. I decided to visit my doctor to see what was happening with my body. He took blood and urine samples to determine my prognosis. The results came back as kidney failure. My kidneys were only operating at 22% and 20% meant dialysis. My urine was full of protein to confirm that my kidneys were dying. I was told that I needed to stop whatever I was doing and drink a lot of water, in which I did. My partying days abruptly ended and I started to take care of myself for awhile.

15 years after my first health scare, I was working as an engineer in a very stagnant job and I balloon up to 283 lbs. I started to feel strange and always winded. I would wake up 8-10 times a night to urinate and I thought I had a prostate problem. So I took a few natural remedies for my prostate, but I still had this issue. So I decided to make an appointment with my doctor. She checked my blood pressure and ordered some blood work. What she discovered was I had heart disease and high cholesterol along with diabetes. She told me I had maybe a year before something major was going to happen, like a heart attack or stroke. I changed my diet and started to exercise. I dropped 93 lbs the right way, through diet and exercise. This life-altering event started my course for writing this book.

Whatever your reason is to change, starting is the hardest part. It is outside our comfort zone. Procrastination and laziness are the most common excuses. Instead of putting it off, make it a priority. You are only hurting yourself by being lazy. Try making your healthy lifestyle fun for your family and friends. Maybe you can introduce some of the things you learned in this book to others. Try making health less of a chore and more pleasurable. It also helps to introduce healthy habits to your loved one in the hopes that they may embrace some of these changes.

Try becoming a good example to others. Show them by example the changes you made to yourself. Don't ever force feed health to an unhealthy person. They tend to rebel and become defensive towards your aggressive stance. Wait until they see the changes you made and some will follow your same path. When they approach you for advice, be loving and understanding. These people are usually very vulnerable and need kind words. Remember when you first started and share your experiences. Have them join you on meal preps and showing them the ropes is another great way to get other involved. Just maybe, you might have found a health buddy.

Our bodies are programmed to eat certain types of addictive foods. This is the reason maintaining a long-term health regimen is so difficult. We become complacent and lazy. We start to give in to unhealthy choices at events and it starts to snowball out of control. A pizza today, a cheeseburger and fries tomorrow and donuts for breakfast can rapidly send your diet off track. We are destined to eat the bad fats, sugar, and salt. Our bodies crave these foods. Is this natural? Our addictive tendencies started with the invention of processed foods.

Heredity also plays a huge role in our food addictions. While in the womb, our mothers probably ate these addictive foods. We learned to crave these ingredients before birth making this addiction a hard habit to break. Change takes a lot of willpower to overcome these addictions. We have to reprogram our taste buds into liking healthy foods since healthy foods don't contain bad fats, sugar, and salt. In order to strive in becoming healthy, we have to take charge of our pleasure centers.

Food is the #1 pleasure center for most humans. When were down and depressed, we turn to food for pleasure, because it is the easiest to satisfy. Try to use another form of pleasure instead, such as laughter or even sex. An occasional "good for the soul" meal won't hurt anyone unless it becomes a habit. Learn to like healthy choices for your pleasure foods. One of my favorite healthy foods is spaghetti squash with marinara sauce. It's healthy and it mimics real spaghetti. Be strict, but not to the point of disliking your food. Only humans eat food for pleasure. All other animals eat food to survive. One of my favorite sayings is "Don't live to eat, eat to live".

Find happiness in other places. If you embrace this philosophy, your journey will become a lot easier. Be strong and this change will be more pleasant. Your addictive foods may change to healthy foods. Unsalted almonds became one of my favorite addictive foods. It used to be potato chip. Our bodies will adapt to whatever we eat.

Change is a healthy part of our lives. Embrace the changes and continue to progress to better yourself. Since we only have one chance on this planet, we should make the most of it. Keep an open mind and try new and exciting adventures to enhance your life. Make changes whenever your life becomes stagnant or unbearable and most of all stay true to yourself. You should be the only judge, no one else.

CHAPTER 3:
Can I Do This?

SELF-DOUBT IS AN insecure thought. Every human questions their abilities on occasions during their lives. Some people let self-doubt control their whole thought process. The "I can't do this" option is a lot easier than exploring your endless possibilities. That's why some people who can climb any mountain and others have trouble convincing themselves to get out of bed. Our brain is our best friend and our worst enemy at the same time. As unbalanced as it may seem for some individuals, most people fall in between. The majority of people seem to be slightly motivated to slightly unmotivated in their lives. The constant teeter totter effect of thoughts and emotions keep them from succeeding, but it keeps their heads above water. The individuals who are always striving for improvement are the highly motivated people and change is normally easy. The population with little motivation and who have trouble caring about themselves are the individuals who need a traumatic event to jump start these severe changes.

Diet is easier to control than exercise. With diet, there is less physical effort involved. If you tend to avoid physical activity, I have good news, this program is 90% diet and 10% exercise. The exercise portion of this diet is optional. Although diet alone allows us to have good health, adding exercise will let us achieve great health. The question is can your brain accept making major dietary changes? This program is designed for longevity, not speed. The changes to your diet will be aggressive, yet gradual. Weaning yourself from bad habits is the easiest way to succeed when you decide to show a commitment. Minimal changes are required over a short period of time to allow you get used to the new diet. Normally a body goes into shock for about 6 weeks because many of our accumulated toxins and chemicals will be released. A person may experience many days of not feeling well.

Our fat cell's stores the majority of the toxins. As you lose weight, the fat is burned as fuel and the toxins will be eliminated by your liver, skin, and kidneys. On some days, the toxins released into our bloodstream become too overwhelming for our system to handle and we may become ill. The symptoms associated with this condition are brain fog, nausea, joint pain, skin eruptions and smelly urine. This condition is called Herxheimer's Syndrome. This is a great condition to experience because it means your body is responding. Some people instantly will stop their diet and say it wasn't for them, without giving it a chance. Most individuals are unaware of the accumulated toxins associated with today's chemical based diets. When you begin to clear out this debris, these toxins will have to be expelled in some manner. Expect these brief initial side effect. These effects go away soon after the start of the diet.

Try to stick to the diet and use your clothes size as your judge. After 6 weeks the body starts to become extremely efficient and welcomes these new changes. The second 6 weeks is like the honeymoon period. You feel great, you're dropping some inches and you have much more energy. The hardest part to overcome is the first 6 weeks. At 12 weeks, the honeymoon period stops and your body will continue repairing itself at a very high rate. With years and years of accumulated toxins, this process may take up to 10 months to clean out much of this debris. This slow, necessary process will keep you away from debilitating health issues in the future.

The exercise portion of the program is mainly for cosmetic purposes, cell rejuvenation and to increase your metabolism. As we age, our calorie usage decreases. To reverse the aging process, we need to increase our metabolism. Exercise can also cause the aging process to accelerate, if not done correctly. If the body gets to the point of absolute exhaustion, our metabolism shuts down. When this condition occurs, our body will try to hibernate. It is human nature to eat a large meal and go to sleep. While we sleep, our metabolism decreases and the big meal we just ate will turn mostly into fat. If we continue doing this routine, we will actually gain weight by over-exercising. The best way to exercise is to work out just to the point of exhaustion. If we don't break the exhaustion threshold, our energy levels will remain high and your metabolism will keep working in high gear. Never use exercise to burn fat, only use exercise for health. This will keep our metabolism running high at all times. As soon as we run out of energy while exercising, we are on our way to hibernation. If we quit exercising before we run out of energy, our body will continue burning calories for the rest of the day. It is pretty simple, don't run out of gas!!!

Do you have what it takes to start this transformation? The Infinity Diet takes dedication to reap all its benefits. If you can find enough motivation to change your health, you can find the time to make it happen. Procrastination won't allow you to lose weight and get healthy. Action will. The question is are you ready to start now, not tomorrow or next year, but now!!! Hopefully, the answer is yes. Today is the best day to start your new life. Here is a fact to help you get motivated, thin people live a lot longer than heavy people. This is very true. Heavy people contract certain illnesses that thin people rarely contract. Some of these diseases are type 2 diabetes, hypertension, high blood pressure and high cholesterol. These illnesses lead to 3 out of the 4 main causes of death, which are a heart attack, stroke, and type 2 diabetes.

All 3 diseases can be reversed on The Infinity Diet. If you have any of these conditions, this may be your incentive to repair ourselves. How about the thought of getting off your medications and having excellent blood work every time you see your doctor? What is easier, taking our meds and feeling bad or feeling great by exercising a little and eating a nutritious diet? You be the judge. The sad part is some people would prefer taking their meds and feeling bad because this type of lifestyle had become normal. Most people are complacent and think this is the only type of life they will ever know, which is not true. A better quality of life is at your fingertips.

Having a highly nutritious diet and proper exercise can repair most of the damage caused by accumulated daily stress. Depending on the person and the amount of damage they accrued the previous day, the degenerative damage can increase the rate of aging. Very little repair is achieved during our awake hours because we are too busy destroying ourselves instead. Our metabolism increases while we sleep to perform the repairs needed from our day's previous damage. On The Infinity Diet, late night snacking is encouraged for repair, but it all depends on what we eat before bed. A bowl of ice cream and some potato chips is discouraged, while an egg or some almonds will aid in our recovery. The key is to recover faster than the damage we create. Almonds or an egg have protein and good fats, while ice cream and potato chip is little more than bad fat and sugar.

Let your health have priority over your cravings. We should eat very low-calorie foods throughout the day to achieve a calorie deficit. There are two reasons we can gain weight by eating fewer calories than your body require. However, normally if we eat less than the required calories, we will lose weight. This will be explained in detail later in this book. The human body defies logic at times. This balancing act between healthy and unhealthy is very difficult for most of us, so don't get discouraged. Remember, we are human after all.

So, do you have the courage to start making good lifestyle changes? Everyone knows complacency and courage can play a huge role in whether we start making changes or not. Can you begin this diet or are you a quitter? Find the courage deep within you and begin this process. The key is to start slow and build your way up. It doesn't have to happen overnight, but it has to happen. It's fine to break away from everyone else to become healthy. Just because people continue their destructive path doesn't mean you have too. By bettering yourself, you will set a wonderful example for other. A salad at the pizza parlor may influence others to try to eat healthy. It takes a lot of effort to change, but if your good eating habits aren't motivation enough for others to follow, so be it. Just take care of yourself. If people ask you about the changes you made, explain this program or better yet, give them this book. Let them decide for themselves. All you can do it give them the tools to succeed. If they don't accept it, at least you tried. Don't preach the program, unless they show interest. It seems to work better for the individuals to come to their own conclusion. If anything is forced upon us, our human nature is to fight or back away. Even if your point is wonderful, most people won't give it chance. If they have the desire to learn more, be their information guide. The success of this book will depend on how many people's lives it may change. If the book only changed your life, it will be a success in this author's eyes.

I hope you found some motivation in the chapter. The mental side of change is difficult and I understand this. I see trainers yell at their clients "Just do it" or by belittling them looking for their motivation. This happens all the time. This may work for some individuals, however, finding motivation by yelling is not enough to encourage others. How do you like to be motivated? I personally like when someone tells me about a positive journey they had encountered. This type of story is very inspirational for me. Health scares, at first were my motivation. Just find what drives you. That's all that manners. A common form of motivation I hear is when individuals want to see their grandchildren grow up. Others have experienced family members who died too early and they don't want to face the same consequences. This diet can help break this genetic pattern. Hopefully, motivation will keep you focused until good habits take over. When your healthy habits become normal, your journey to great health will become a maintenance program. When you have reached this plateau, you have succeeded.

CHAPTER 4:
How Did We Get Here?

BEFORE THE INDUSTRIAL AGE, people ate fresh foods which contained no pollutants. Soon after, chemicals started to be introduced to our systems through food, air, and water. We absorb these chemicals and store many of these toxins in our liver, bones and fat cells. In the beginning, only small amounts of these toxins were present. However, as time passes, more chemicals were being introduced, so our bodies had to adapt to the influx of pollutants in our environment. When the pharmaceutical companies took over the medical schools in the 1920's, an increase in chemical based medications were introduced to the public. Drugs became commonplace as treatments for most illnesses. The chemical industry started to discredit the holistic healing practices as quackery, at this time. Therefore, chemical based drugs became the norm instead of natural remedies. Many of the chemical companies transformed into pharmaceutical companies, because of the huge profits associated with this newly created industry. New legislation was also introduced to make healing or curing illegal. The term "cure" was banned from all doctor's offices and hospitals and its use is punishable by law. Therefore, holistic doctors were curing and healing, while the pharmaceutical doctors were treating. Many holistic doctors were sent to prison for curing people, eliminating their practices. This began the birth of the chemical medicine monopoly.

Few people had cancer or diabetes a few hundred years ago. Most people were healthy. Nature intended for us to eat natural foods. Take a look at the labels in the grocery stores. What you'll find is a bunch of words that are unrecognizable. These are usually the chemicals in our foods. How many more chemicals can our bodies endure? The answer is NO MORE CHEMICALS!!! Look at the illnesses our children are contacting today. Children rarely had illnesses such as cancer, diabetes, autism, obesity, and ADHD 30 years ago. Today, in 2017, I personally know three children with cancer. As a society, we have to eliminate these chemical laced products by not purchasing them. Our health is more important than the profit margins of Big Business.

Our food supply is designed to taste good yet make us sick. Let's take a look at breakfast cereal for an example. Children eat tons of this junk every day. Cereal is basically a little protein and a whole lot of simple carbs (simple carbs turn directly into sugar or is sugar to start with). Oh, did I forget, and little-added vitamins and minerals to make it sound attractive to the parents. If your cereal has fortified iron, I would strongly recommend looking for another breakfast for your children. Recent studies have shown that fortified iron combined with animal protein and calcium (milk) greatly increases our chances of getting arterial sclerosis. This makes breakfast cereal the perfect concoction to lead to all of today's heart issues.

It's also no wonder why our children have become such behavioral issues in the morning. If milk and cereal are combined, this makes the perfect formula for hyperactivity. Milk is primarily fat and sugar with a bunch of dead bacteria and some protein. The last paragraph explained what cereal is made from a bunch of sugar. How would you feel drinking 3 soft drinks before work? That's what millions of children are getting for breakfast. This meal puts a heavy load on their pancreas to produce insulin and sometimes it can't keep up. Now, these children are on their way to diabetes. If the cereal is made from corn, beet sugar, soy, cottonseed or canola oil, it probably has GMO (genetically modified organisms) ingredients. GMO ingredients have been linked to food allergies, severe intestinal issues and sterility, just to name a few. Just think how much larger this picture gets since we only examined breakfast cereal. What else are we eating the rest of the day? Think about it.

This author is convinced everything we eat has a man-made chemical in its composition. From our breakfast cereals to homegrown tomatoes, nothing is left untouched. The tomatoes get hit with air pollution through its skin and through the roots. The water is full of chlorine and fluoride. Both chemicals are highly poisonous and can cause many medical issues including thyroid problems and bone loss. Think about it, why do we need fluoride to eat our tooth enamel away? Common sense would tell you to let it grow. I know people who never use fluoride toothpaste and they rarely have dental issues. My daughter and I stopped using fluoride toothpaste 5 years ago and our teeth have been fine ever since, even though we both have genetically thin tooth enamel. Since stopping the use of fluoride toothpaste, we have had sparkling check-ups every dental visit.

What can society do about the chemical problem? We have to constantly rid our bodies of these toxins and ingest the cleanest possible air, food, and water. The best way is to buy organic foods or plant your own garden. Maybe you can find others who would like to get involved and start an urban garden. The health benefits are tremendous by eating our own produce. A number of farmer's only farmer's markets are starting to pop up. Some of the vendors at farmer's markets are buying cases of non-organic produce and reselling their items as organic. Look for the organic label, before purchasing such items. Soak your produce in vinegar or ozonated water to rid your food of these unwanted pesticides. We will talk more about ozonated water in the following chapter. Ozonated water releases the chemicals and pesticides from your produce and sterilizing the food at the same time.

Understanding food composition can be complicated and confusing. Let's have a small lesson of this complex subject. The hardest group to understand is carbohydrates or carbs, for short. Carbs basically fit 3 categories, simple carbs, complex carbs, and fiber. Simple carbs are the sugars and foods that can easily turn into sugar. Some examples of simple carbs are cane and beet sugar, corn syrup, milk sugar, potatoes and all enriched grain foods like white bread, white rice, and pasta. The best way to tell if a food is a simple carb is to leave it in your mouth for 30 seconds. If the item becomes sweet, this food must be a simple carb. Simple carbs start to breakdown in our saliva, therefore transforming into sugar before it reaches our stomach. When eaten, these sugars have to be utilized right away or they will turn directly into fat. People dependent on simple carbs tends to be overweight and have to eat more frequently to satisfy their hunger.

A complex carbohydrate is a time released sugar. It takes our digestive system up to 4 hours to process these foods into energy. These carbs include all the veggies, fruits, and whole grains. The lowest calorie of these carbs is vegetables. Veggies are very high in nutrients and very low on calories. This makes vegetables the backbone of The Infinity Diet. Fruit is basically veggies with sugar and by weight, they tend to carry twice the calories compared to vegetables. Fruit is also approved on The Infinity Diet. Fiber is basically non-digestible foods that help transport waste matter out of the digestive system. Examples of fiber rich foods are beans, vegetables, certain fruits and whole grains. Fiber dense foods are approved on The Infinity Diet, except for the highly dense whole grains. Whole grains carry more calories than the fruit and veggies due to the density of these foods. The excessive calories belonging to whole grains outweigh the benefit associated with the fiber. Underneath the fiber and complex carbs, the true core of whole grains is simple carbs.

Fats are also very confusing to understand. Fat is the most calorie-dense food, yet necessary for optimal health in The Infinity Diet. Good fats are essential for brain function, cell replication and keeping our circulatory system functioning correctly. The bad fats are the absolute opposite of the good fats by causing damage to this vital life sustaining systems. Some of the good fats are olive oil, flaxseed oil, coconut oil, avocados and nuts (not peanuts). Some of the bad fats are margarine, corn oil, cottonseed oil, soybean oil and canola oil. Animal fats are both good and bad at the same time. They tend to clog our circulatory system, but have many of the good fat properties as well. The key to consuming animal fat is to eat it in moderation. Many of the bad fats are also GMO products, which can lead to severe health issues. Try to avoid fried foods from unknown sources. Many restaurants use the cheapest and the least healthy oils in their fryers.

Body fat is our energy reserve during lean times. Unfortunately, most people eat low nutrient foods and our body believes it is going to starve. Therefore, the body stores fat to preserve life. In general, people eat too many calories, without eating enough nutrients. Any calories leftover from the day turns directly into fat. A calorie deficit during the day turns your body fat into energy. It's a checks and balance game associated with weight gain and weight loss.

Protein is used strictly for muscle function. Each person has their own protein requirement based on their body composition. A 5-year-old girl may need 20 grams of protein to maintain her muscle function, while a 260 lbs body builder may need 350 grams of protein to maintain his. There is little energy associated with protein, so protein is strictly a recovery food. The best way to calculate your protein needs is to track your diet. The majority of people consume too much protein. Excessive protein consumption has been linked to osteoporosis and kidney issues. Try to keep your protein consumption low until you experience muscle weakness and then slowly increase your intake until you find the right balance for your body composition.

Vitamins, minerals and other necessary nutrients are found mainly in fresh foods. The majority of processed foods add artificial nutrients to counteract the loss of the natural nutrients being stripped away during processing. The food companies use this health propaganda to help sell their products to consumers. If we eat nutritious foods, our body will be satisfied and our excessive body fat can be used as energy. The body will never starve as long an abundance of nutrients are being consumed. When you reduce your body fat content down to around 10%, your body may trigger a warning that too little calories remain, which can tell your brain to consume more food.

One of the main causes of weight gain and poor health is the overuse of sugar in most our foods. When the food industry turned corn into sugar, corn syrup became the desired ingredient in almost everything produced. Bread, salad dressing, soft drinks, and ketchup are just among the few foods using corn based sugar in their ingredients. Along with sugar, many of our foods consist of grains and grain-based oils, such as breakfast cereals, tortilla chips, cookies, crackers, and bread. If we don't use the calories associated with these foods immediately, our body will store the leftover calories as fat. The combination of simple sugars and bad fats is a wonderful recipe for a diabetic disaster, especially if we add salt to this mix. Most of our population overindulges on these life-threatening foods. Let's look at a sample diet.

Breakfast	Lunch	Dinner
(2) Pancakes	Cheeseburger	Spaghetti w/Marinara
(2) Fried Eggs	French Fries	Zucchini w/ Stewed Tomatoes
(3) Bacon	Coke	Garlic Bread w/ Margarine
(2) Toast w/Margarine		(2) Glasses of Wine
Coffee		

Breakfast: Pancakes are flour (simple carb), sugar, eggs (good), milk (fat and sugar) and cooked with vegetable oil (bad fat). Eggs (good) are cooked in vegetable oil (bad fat) and maybe salt and pepper (good). Bacon is protein (good) and good/bad fat. The toast is flour (simple carb), yeast, salt, and water. The margarine is 100% cell destroying trans fats. The eggs come from chickens fed with hormones and GMO feed. The vegetable oils are usually from a GMO plant. The bacon is from a pig that probably ate nothing but GMO food all its life. The milk is probably from a cow that is fed GMO feed. The ingredients are very high in sugar from the toast and pancakes. The eggs and bacon provide a good source of protein. The coffee is a diuretic and it dehydrates the body.

Lunch: The cheeseburger has flour (simple carbs), yeast, salt, beef (protein & good/ fat), lettuce (complex carb), tomato (complex carb), onion (complex carb), pickles (complex carb and salt), dressing (salt and sugar) and cheese (bad fat and salt). The fries are potatoes (simple carb), salt and vegetable oil (bad fat). The Coke is sugar, chemicals, and water. The beef and cheese are probably from cows that were fed GMO feed. Although beef fat is good for our cells, it is bad for our circulatory system. The oil in the fries is made from corn, canola, cottonseed, and soy, or a combination of several. All of these oils usually come from GMO-based plants.

Dinner: The spaghetti is made from wheat flour (simple carb), water and salt. The marinara sauce is tomatoes (complex carb), sugar, water and a bunch of spices that tend to be very good for you. The zucchini and stewed tomatoes are both complex carbs with some salt. The garlic bread has flour (simple carb), garlic (complex carb), yeast, salt and water and the margarine is pure cell destroying garbage. The wine's alcohol turns directly into a simple sugar with an increased amount of calories. Let's call alcohol a Super Simple Sugar. Almost all wine uses chemicals as preservatives. Margarine and zucchini are the hidden GMO products in this meal. Yes, zucchini is now a GMO product, along with Mexican papaya, some apples, and plums.

This normal daily diet can be a nightmare for your body. Let's break it down. The worst ingredients for your health are the sugars, grains and bad fats. Since the invention of processed foods in the 1950's, the food manufacturers began introducing various simple carbs, excessive salt and trans fats in our diets. The food manufacturers knew these foods were very addictive and inexpensive to produce. Their invention was intended to increase profits for the food manufacturers and the medical industry alike. This diet basically invented type 2 diabetes and our population's health has been on a steady decline ever since. The health care industry had to create new drugs to combat these issues associated with this diet. If you analyze this sample diet objectively; this should be a wake-up call to anyone who cares about self-preservation.

The conclusion regarding our sample diet is there are too many simple carbs, salt, bad oils and GMO ingredients. These foods are associated with weight gain and a great number of health issues. GMO foods have been known to destroy the little hair like fibers call villi in our intestines. These fibers absorb the nutrients from our digesting food and transport them to our pancreas. If these fibers are destroyed, our bodies become nutrient deficient and this condition leads to Celiac disease. If we eat non-nutritious foods or our food is not being properly absorbed, our brains keep sending signals to eat, even if our stomachs are full. This condition causes over-eating, obesity, and malnutrition.

Our biggest concern is how to stop ingesting chemicals. There are currently 84,000 different chemicals being manufactured. Many of these chemicals are used in our food and prescription drugs or are leached into the air and water supply. Just in the GMO foods alone, it seems to be impossible to avoid these chemicals. Studies have shown that GMO foods can cause severe digestive disorders, such as gluten sensitivity, food allergies, Celiac and Crohn's disease along with severe reproductive issues. Practically all animals used for consumption are fed with GMO feed and the majority of frying oils are originated from GMO plants. Ultimately, we can't trust the food manufacturers to supply us with safe food.

When we eat out, we are subjected to a variety of low-cost ingredients being used in our foods. Can we 100% control the quality of foods we consume? The answer is no. There are too many booby traps standing in our way to proper health. We would have to grow our own food or move to a country that banned the use of all GMO foods. There are 38 such countries worldwide, as of this writing. These countries care more about their citizens than the money. If more and more countries join this ban, humanity may have a chance. With the way GMO foods are damaging the male reproductive organs, children will not be conceived outside of a laboratory in the near future.

However, the other chemicals will still exist. Just the plastic alone used to preserve our food is enough to cause health issues. We have reached the point of no return. The only solution is to detoxify ourselves on a continuous basis and to stop eating GMO foods.

Our addictive, low nutrient food supply is less of the problem than our willpower. People are generally weak when it comes to their tastes. I believe if quality foods were more available and reasonably priced, people would eat better. This is evident in Europe. Most of the continent maintains healthy food sources and it shows in the condition of their citizens. The majority of the population is height-weight proportionate. This means that their weight matches a healthy ratio based on their height. For instance, a male at 5'10", should weigh between 149-183 lbs to meet this ratio. Does your body fit into this 34 lbs gap? Anyway, people regarded as height-weight proportionate are considered healthy. Another example is a 5'2" woman should weigh between 99-121 lbs. Anything over this maximum weight is considered overweight. Double the weight window and that becomes obesity. For instance, if the same woman was 22 lbs heavier than her maximum height-weight proportion, she would be considered obese at 143 lbs. The 5'10" man would be obese at 217 lbs based on the ratio of adding 34 lbs over his maximum height-weight proportion numbers.

These numbers can be incorrect based on certain genetic variations or by exercise. This author had a body builder friend, who was 5'5" and 255 lbs. His height-weight proportion ratio should be between 122-150 lbs. According to the numbers, this made him 105 lbs overweight, yet he had only 7% body fat. His total body fat was only 18 lbs. If you are muscular, the ratios may vary.

The main question is can we reverse the damage created by our bad diet? The answer is yes. If we decide to eat natural foods, we will become healthier. The real question is can we do it? Our diet, as a society, is horrible. Some major behavioral changes will have to take place. What is our food other than calories and nutrients? It's a pleasure in a non-pleasurable world. I hope people can find more enjoyable outlets and less pleasure associated with food.

It's possible to dedicate an hour a day for meal prepping to remain healthy. If you have a garden, it's possible to dedicate even more time to maintain your health. Consider finding a partner who can help you plan your meals. Become creative and make your diet a priority. We only have one chance to live on this planet, so why waste it.

It's possible to eat 30 years off your life. Isn't that a lot to lose? How about the idea of increasing your life span by 30 years instead? Doesn't that sound better? Both are possible. Short of getting into a car accident, it's possible to live a high-quality life until we choose not to live anymore. Which path will you choose? Most of us are in the middle. With the food and drug industries working against our health, our chances of maintaining a high quality of life into our twilight years are now highly unlikely.

Who do you blame for your weight issues? This author lost 94 lbs himself, so I qualify. I blamed my job, instead of placing the blame on myself. I had a sit-down job as a design engineer. My bosses would continually bring me great lunches because I made more money for the company the longer I sat behind my desk. I had high blood pressure, high cholesterol, and diabetes. Most of the blame should be pinned on us with a little of the blame going to the food industry.

It takes effort to eat healthy and it appears laziness is the root cause to eat unhealthily. Most people refuse to cook after a long day at work. Fast meals have become the norm. Typically, the faster the food is prepared, the worse it is for us. Fried foods and ramen noodles can be made fast and are horrible for our bodies. Most burgers are now microwaved at fast food restaurants and this author knows of one restaurant chain serving pre-cooked foods from plastic bags. The bag is placed into boiling water until the contents are hot. Just imagine the chemicals being leached into our bodies from these hot plastics. The contents are then poured onto a plate and decorated to look appetizing. In this instance, a restaurant isn't preparing our food, a factory is. Home cooked meals are guaranteed to be fresh and healthy if you know how to cook. Cooking can be fun and easy for the whole family if you allow it. This book dedicates a chapter to food preparation with several great healthy recipes.

CHAPTER 5:
I Thought This Was A Diet Book!!!

THIS DIET IS DIFFERENT than most diets. It combines many facets of other successful diets into one. The most critical part of this diet is converting our bodies to burn fat more readily than carbohydrates. If we look at our bodies, we have fat everywhere. The fat is attached to our skin and collects around our liver. If we peeled off our skin, everyone would appear to look the same, lean muscle, bones and organs. Our bodies contain about 280,000,000 fats cells, with the majority of the fat cells attached to our skin. These cells are like sponges, but instead of absorbing water, these cells collect fat and toxins. If we increase our calorie intake, our body will store the unused calories as fat. This fat is collected to be used as future energy. If we use more calories than we consume, our body will take the stored fat and convert it into energy. By converting our main fuel source to fat instead of carbs, our body will depend on the fat for fuel. If we have a calorie deficit on a given day, our body may pull the energy needed to survive from your thighs, butt, and belly. Whether we digest it or it's hanging from our arms, our body sees fat in the same light. Fat is just fat.

Treat your food intake like a bank account, but in reverse. The unused calories from your day will turn into fat, which constitutes a deposit. Therefore, a calorie deficit on a given day will become a withdrawal. So if we eat fewer calories than what we use, we lose fat. It's all checks and balances. This is ultimately why people become overweight. They eat more calories than they burn. This is the truth with all diets. This portion of the Infinity Diet is no different. This book explains how the body works based on science and how to burn the most calories possible while eating natural foods. That's right, no supplements. Supplements are laden with chemicals and the purpose of this book is to rid ourselves of unwanted chemicals. The Infinity Diet is designed to maintain a healthy height-weight proportion and great health until we determine our own finish line.

Our body likes to use carbohydrates for energy because carbs turn easily to sugar. With fat, our liver has to work very hard to convert this source into energy. It takes a couple of weeks to retrain our bodies to depend on this alternate fuel source. This fat utilizing diet will increase your metabolism because it takes an extra amount of energy to turn fat into sugar.

Replacing our sugar based diet with vegetable based complex carbs and good fat is the next step. Like explained earlier, complex carbs take several hours to digest. This makes complex carbs time released energy. By spreading out the distribution of sugar over a longer period of time, our bodies have to search for an alternate energy source. When our body starts to realize our main fuel source isn't sugar, an avocado or some almonds begin to look very appetizing to our bodies. The hardest part is getting your body trained to burn fat as its primary fuel source.

Ever since birth, we were raised on a sugar based diet. From breast milk to baby cereal, sugar has been our main source of energy. On the other hand, the Eskimos depend on seals and fish for survival. Seals and fish contain no carbs, just fat and protein. The Eskimos happen to be the leanest people on this planet as a population. What should this information tell you? In order to become lean, should we eat like Eskimos? Not entirely. The Eskimos experience some vitamin deficiencies because of their limited diet. We don't want our bodies to become entirely dependent on fat as our only fuel source. However, a large portion of our diet should use fat as its main source of energy.

To regulate our weight loss, we can increase our carb intake to slow the fat burning process. This diet is like having a gas pedal, the harder you push, the faster you go. If you lose too much weight and the skin appears to sag, introduce more carbs into your diet. Maybe a small bowl of rice or a tortilla a day should slow down the fat burning process enough to allow the skin to rebound. Our skin does heal. However, it takes time and the right nutrients for our skin to tighten. Stretch marks are permanent, but our unwanted skin will heal and become tight again after about 4 years if we remain on a veggie based diet. Most dark green leafy vegetables are high in anti-oxidants and collagen. These nutrients are essential for healthy skin. Just remember, it took years to become unhealthy, so it takes time for our bodies to regain our health once more. Humans are very resilient creatures. We can heal relatively fast.

Another important part of this diet is to eat highly nutritious foods. Most of today's diet is full of calories but contain little nutrients. If we replace our calorie dense foods with nutritious foods, our bodies will also use fat as its primary fuel source. Our body only cares about nutrients because it stores plenty of calories in our thighs, butt, and abdomen. This is another way for our bodies to utilize fat as energy. The most nutritious and readily available food is fruit and vegetables. Produce is available at the local farmer's market or store year-round. Make sure to clean your produce thoroughly due to the use of pesticides. Washing the produce in a vinegar solution or ozonated water is a few of the ways to eliminate the impurities from your produce. If you can find organic produce, buy it. Try to eat the lowest amount of chemicals as possible. The best source is having our own garden. This way you can guarantee the purity and freshness of your food supply.

Another excellent source of nutrient dense food is nuts. Almonds, walnuts, cashews, and macadamia nuts, plus many others, are all high in good fat, protein, fiber and a host of other nutrients. For example, Brazil nuts are extremely high in one of the most powerful anti-oxidants known called Selenium. This mineral is very important for thyroid function and is great for preventing cancer. Men have to be careful using this mineral because an overabundance of Selenium can shut down their prostate function, causing sexual and urination issues. Peanuts come from legume family, therefore are not considered a nut. Peanuts are closely related to peas and beans. Try to avoid salted nuts. The salt is very high in sodium, which can cause circulatory and cell issues plus excessive water retention. Large amounts of water in your blood can cause high blood pressure and heart issues.

On a vegetable based diet, a lack of protein can become a concern. Protein is essential for muscle rejuvenation and function. As explained earlier, each individual needs their own specific protein requirement based on their body composition. Since most vegetables are low in protein, other foods have to be eaten to satisfy our muscle requirements. Legumes, seeds, and nuts all are excellent sources of protein and fiber. Grains are also a source of protein and fiber; however, grains are calorie and carbohydrate dense and should be limited. Remember, we are changing our bodies to burn fat, not carbs. The abundance of carbohydrates in grains outweighs the benefits of the protein in these foods. Nuts are a much better source of protein and are high in good fat.

The health issues related to eating gluten protein has become tremendous. This author recommends eliminating gluten entirely from the diet. The food industry has altered the wheat plant to produce a short and sturdier version for more profitability. Yesterday's wheat grew to about 6 feet high and was very fragile. Today's plants are about 3 feet tall and stocky to withstand high winds and to increase the yield. Due to the genetic changes to this grain, we are no longer able to digest the gluten protein associated with this plant. The current gluten protein is similar to sandpaper in our intestines. With our GMO induced digestive issues, gluten increases the damage already created by these modified foods. If we consider the villi in our intestines being eaten away by the GMO foods and adding gluten based sandpaper to our intestines, what do we get? That's right, a mess. Sooner than later, we will become malnourished. When we become malnourished, our bodies tell us to eat. So we eat and eat and eat more of these calorie-dense foods like pizza and French fries to make up for the lost nutrients our bodies are looking for. But where are the nutrients? Can we even process the nutrients, if we happen to eat them? The answer is no. Our bodies are taking in too many calories searching for nutrients, which cause a calorie overload. This literally is a GROWING problem. This author believes the majority of people will have to receive their nutrients by other means by 2030. Sublingual (under the tongue) and skin absorbed nutrients along with injections will become the norm. Although the human body can live from the sun's nutrients and water for up to 6 months, I believe our population will become very unhealthy in the near future. Do you want to be like the rest of the population?

Animal proteins are both beneficial and risky, at the same time. The biggest risk associated with eating animal based proteins is the meat is very acidic and most animals are fed GMO feed. Hormones are also added to increase the yield, with many of these animals. Antibiotics are also given to the animals to prevent illness. These antibiotics have caused humans to create an immunity to many other drugs. Animal proteins include all the meats, eggs, cheese and dairy products. As for a healthy meat source, lamb only feed on grass for their dietary needs and they tend to be the healthiest of all the animals we consume. The main health benefit from eating meat is meat is a slow digesting protein. Meat supplies nutrients to our muscles for a couple of days while it runs through our digestive system. This steady flow of protein is great for athletes and growing individuals. Animal protein also contains all the essential amino acids. Amino acids are broken down from the proteins and are transported to the muscles for recovery. Protein does not go directly into the muscles. The amino acids do.

Out of all the animal proteins available, eggs are the healthiest. Eggs are very high in cholesterol and contain 8 grams of protein along with many other nutrients. People associate cholesterol as being unhealthy because everyone is misled to its importance for our survival. If we are healthy, eating foods with high cholesterol won't matter. Cholesterol protects our circulatory system from tears and aneurysms, which can cause strokes or heart attacks. Most people who have cholesterol issues also have damaged circulatory systems. Our liver is like a plumber. When we have a leak in our circulatory system, the liver dispatched cholesterol to patch the holes. If we have too many holes to be patched up, we get cholesterol build up in these damaged areas. The most effective way to prevent cholesterol blockages is to change our diet. The tears are caused by hardened calcium in our circulatory system. When the calcium solidifies and gets dislodged, tears can occur. If the tear is too large, a clot can form and cause a stroke. The Infinity Diet can eliminate many of these potentially fatal events from occurring. If your family has a predisposition to heart-related issues through heredity, this diet should be a big part of your life. We only have one chance on this planet, why not get the most out of it.

Small fish are a very good source of protein and other nutrients. These small fish contain Omega 3 oil, which is essential for proper liver function and to normalize cholesterol levels in our blood. Fish is also high in iodine. Iodine is essential in cell rejuvenation, radiation elimination and thyroid function. A high number of our population is iodine deficient. If our thyroid isn't functioning correctly, our metabolism, heart rate, and many other vital functions are affected

Large fish pose a health risk due to the potential of contracting mercury poisoning. The general rule is the larger the fish, the higher the mercury levels. Mercury poisoning is caused by fossil fuel and coal pollution in our water supply. Small organisms have taken a liking to this pollution. When the little fish eat these organisms, nothing happens. But when the small fish eat the little fish, the process starts to change into mercury. The small fish are still safe to eat. However, when the medium fish eats the small fish and the big fish eats the medium fish, the original pollution from the organisms' changes into mercury. Mercury poisoning is very common with frequent fish eaters. Mothers who eat fish during pregnancy carry their mercury poisoning onto their young, as explained earlier.

Crabs, lobsters and other bottom feeding sea creatures should not be consumed. Many of these creatures eat the pollutants which settle to the bottom of the ocean. Pacific lobsters now have an appetite for oil sludge leaked by offshore oil drilling rigs. Remember, whatever the animals eat, we eat it too. Recently, genetically modified salmon were introduced into our food supply. These fish grow at an alarming rate to twice the size of a normal salmon. The facts aren't out on the possible health issues created by this GMO fish.

Poultry is a wonderful source of protein and nutrients and is lower in fat than other animal products. Unfortunately, this author has to question the adaptation of the chicken. The food industry has changed the genetics of the chicken to be harvested in 1/4 of the required time and to grow huge breasts. The food industry markets this creature as an all-natural chicken. A real natural chicken is a small animal that normally lives about 6 months before harvesting, instead of 6 weeks. Form your own opinion. Eating free range chicken or turkey is your best bet to avoid any genetic tampering. The normal diet for turkeys and chickens is greens, worms, and insects, not GMO corn.

When it comes to consuming beef, this author feels the harm outweighs the good. Though a good protein source, commercial beef is too risky to eat because of the artificial hormones and antibiotics which are given to the cattle. The risk of contracting salmonella or E-coli has increased tremendously due to the cattle's GMO corn and soy diet. The growth hormones given to the cattle are direct cancer-causing agents which are banned from the rest of the world, except for Canada and the United States. These countries are not allowed to export their beef because of the use of these chemicals. The slaughtered beef are now dipped into a selenium bath to try to combat the likelihood of people contracting cancer from these chemicals. We have to endure all these health risks so the cattle can become 60 lbs heavier with less fat and be slaughtered 2 weeks earlier in the name of increased profits.

Pigs will eat anything. This is scary since we eat them. This is the reason why pork meat needs to be cooked thoroughly. Pork overall is a good source of protein. Although pork fat is very salty by nature, it is better to consume than beef fat. Again, do we know what we're eating? The answer is no. A major food chain who advertises organic food had to pull pork off their menu for this very reason. I believe the majority of pork in unsatisfactory for human consumption because of the strong likelihood of these animal eating GMO-based feed.

Australian or New Zealand lamb is a good source of animal protein. These animals are grass fed and raised in a non-GMO environment. If you are able to locate this product, The Infinity Diet allows the consumption of this meat.

Fat comes in many different forms. From lard to coconut oil, fat is the most complex of all the foods we consume. The public has been brainwashed into thinking fat is the cause of our overweight population. This is only partially true. We have low-fat or non-fat versions of various products throughout our grocery stores. Our body actually requires fat for proper health, but only good fat. The individuals who restrict their diets of fat will experience severe health issues. Fat is needed for brain and joint function and to produce bile, which is essential for digestion and the absorption of fat-soluble vitamins. Therefore, fat plays an important role in our health. Since the topic of fat is so confusing to most of the population who aren't physicists, I will break down the fats and tell how they affect our health. The most important fat is the long chain fatty acids and coconut oil. Each of these fats plays a key role in proper health.

The most important are the oils high in Omega 3 fatty acids. The Omega 3 rich oils are fish oil, cod liver oil, and flax seed oil. These oils are critical for heart health. Omega 3 fatty acid helps reduce calcium buildup in our circulatory system and lowers our blood pressure by normalizing our cholesterol levels. These acids also increase the speed in which our blood flows through our system. This is very important considering the faster our blood travels, the higher our metabolism is increased.

The Omega 6 fatty acids come from various sources such as vegetable oils, poultry, seeds, and nuts. These acids aid in our brain function, bone health, reproductive health, hair growth, regulation of metabolism and help produce a hormone essential for blood clotting. Individuals should only consume 50% of the Omega 6 fatty acids compared to Omega 3 fatty acids. No more than 15% of our total dietary calories should come from Omega 6's. If we consume over 15% of our dietary intake, we subject ourselves to numerous health issues such as inflammatory conditions like rheumatoid arthritis, asthma, cardiovascular diseases and much more. Much of our population consume as high as a 25 to 1 ratio in favor of Omega 6's over the Omega 3's in today's diet. This out of balance ratio is one of the many reasons we experience poor health.

Most solid fats are saturated fats and should be limited in your diet. These fats include red meat, milk related products, coconut oil, cheese and many of the oils used in the baking process. In moderation, these fats do little harm to bodies and are excellent for cell rejuvenation. To maintain our health, up to 10% of our calories can come from such fats. Most people overindulge with these products, especially in the meat and cheese department. A recent study revealed that saturated fat does little harm to our cholesterol levels and to the buildup of plaque. The majority of damage is caused by increasing our body weight from eating too many calories and the ability of saturated fat to store toxins. As we eat the animal's fat toxins, our liver, kidneys and lymphatic system have to process all these extra undesirables. Try to eat grain fed meats as much as possible, since these animals seem to be healthier and less contaminated than commercial animals.

Coconut oil is unique compared to all the other fats. This wonderful oil is the only fat that starts to breakdown in our saliva and turns directly into energy. This makes coconut oil one of the best fuels for our body. By converting to a fat dependent diet, coconut oil can supply energy for long periods of time, which makes it very desirable for endurance athletes. If clean energy is needed, coconut oil is the best choice.

Coconut oil also can't be stored in our bodies, so this oil will not increase our body weight. This unique oil also has the ability to boost our metabolism by means of being harder to digest. Although coconut oil is a saturated fat outside our body, this oil becomes an unsaturated fat within our body. Coconut oil becomes liquid at 76 degrees. The Infinity Diet recommends coconut oil to be used for any desired application. Since coconuts have so many wonderful nutrients, a person can survive on coconuts alone. This author believes that nature put coconut trees on most small islands because of this very reason.

Trans fats are to blame for many of our population's health problems beginning in the 1950's. These fats are synthetic oils produced to increase profits for the food industry. The food industry discovered that oil could be modified to last longer by introducing hydrogen to its contents, which turned liquid oil into a solid. Margarine is a prime example of a trans fat. This fat causes many health issues from cell damage to increasing our bad cholesterol and decreasing our good cholesterol. Although trans fats are being eliminated slowly from our food supply, they still exist in many processed goods. Read the ingredients first before purchasing your food. If you see hydrogen in the ingredients, don't buy it. Even small amounts of trans fats will cause damage to our bodies. We can still find trans fats in many of our baked and fried goods. Remember when we eat out, we have no idea what we're eating.

Fresh pressed juices are wonderful beverages with so many positive attributes, yet few negative issues. These juices are packed with an abundance of nutrients and our bodies usually absorb these nutrients extremely well. Pressed juices hold their nutrients much longer than the standard centrifugal juices made at home or at low-end juice bars. When the juice is pressed, the nutrients remain longer because there is no heat involved during the juicing process. The normal shelf life is about three days for pressed juices, while centrifugal produced juices last about 10 minutes before their nutrients are lost. Centrifugal produced juices are made with tremendous speed from the machine, which creates heat. When food is heated, a great deal of the original nutrients is lost.

Pre-packaged juices are nutritious but have been pasteurized to maintain a long shelf life. The pasteurization process requires the juice to be briefly heated to kill any living organisms within the juice. This process creates dead food. When it comes to eating, live foods are much more nutritious. Unfortunately, most people rely on dead food in their diets. The definition of a live food is if it came from the earth or lived as a creature of the earth. This pretty much means fruits, vegetables, and animals. All other foods are considered dead and depending on processing, stripped of its nutritional value during manufacturing. Therefore, raw foods are typically the most nutritious items we can eat.

Many of us like to drink alcohol for various reasons. From social and recreational purposes to addiction, alcohol is the drug of choice for most. Alcohol is very calorie dense, with 7 calories per gram or 198 calories per ounce. Only fat is higher at 9 calories per gram. This poison can't be stored in our bodies and our body tries to eliminate this beverage through our liver and kidneys as fast as possible. During this process, our body's only purpose is to rid the alcohol out of our system. This affects our insulin levels since our body will not regulate our blood sugar during the elimination process. Normally heavy drinkers will get severe blood sugar spikes and levels of extremely low blood sugar. This condition, over a period of time, causes severe medical issues with their liver and pancreas.

If you have ever noticed if you drink while dancing or playing softball your muscles feel tired? Alcohol is dependant of sugar, so it drains the sugar storage out of our muscles during exercise. Over time, insulin becomes ineffective towards the breakdown of the sugars and can cause for diabetes. Alcohol will also severely dehydrate you. When we consume alcohol, our body decreases a hormone that helps regulate water.

If alcohol is consumed, please drink in moderation. Moderation means 1 drink a day for a small or elderly person and 2 drinks for a larger person. There are some actual health benefits with drinking alcohol in moderation. It may decrease your risk of heart disease, strokes, and diabetes if practiced in moderation. If you don't consume alcohol presently, it is not advisable to drink for health purposes. The damage it causes is more severe than the good it does for our body. If you currently drink, consider the harm versus the benefit that may occur with prolonged use. Maybe this fact will detour you from indulging in this beverage. Alcohol should not be consumed on The Infinity Diet.

When it comes to eating or drinking dairy, this author feels the products produced from cow's milk should not be ingested, except for one product introduced later in this book. Cows should drink cow milk, not humans. Cow's milk is extremely hard to digest and most people are becoming less tolerance to these products. If we consume any dairy, the dairy should come from an animal very close to our own DNA, such as a goat, a sheep, or better yet, a human. The only reason we have cow dairy products is because cows produce a lot of milk and it's profitable. There is no other reason. The public has been brainwashed by the media to believe that dairy is good for us. Today's milk is basically dead bacteria, sugar (lactose), a little protein and water. Cows have been engineered to produce milk with little nutritional value. This allows the milk to be fortified with artificial calcium and vitamin D to appear to be healthy for human consumption.

Humans are the only mammals on this planet that eat or drink dairy products after being weaned off our mother's milk. If you choose to consume dairy-like products, look for other options. Almond milk and coconut milk are wonderful alternatives. Both of these products are wonderful for consumption. Coconut milk is the best alternative since it contains all the vital electrolytes and many other nutrients.

Soy milk should also be avoided because this milk has the ability to shut down our thyroid function and is high in human growth hormone, which can cause havoc for individuals with cancer and inflammatory diseases such as rheumatoid arthritis. Soy is also a female based plant and it should not be consumed by men. It can cause such conditions as lowered testosterone, decreased sperm production and gynecomastia or male enlarged breasts. Other female based products to avoid is beer made from hops and Marijuana based products. Many of our fried foods and salad dressings also contain soybean oil. The majority of this oil is derived from GMO plants. The hormones associated with this oil are very likely causing the feminizing of today's men. Their sexual organs are now under attack by the food industries.

The healthiest beverage of any sort is water. Our bodies contain around 75% water by volume and it's the only liquid we need for survival. The benefits associated with drinking water is countless. From regulating our blood pressure to cleaning out our kidneys, water is the one essential element needed for survival. Like explained earlier, a person can live up to 6 months on sun and water, but a person usually can't live for more than 3 days without this life-sustaining beverage.

Out of all the different waters available, freshly ozonated water is far superior to any of the other varieties. In Europe, ozone gas is infused into the water supply to disinfect the water of unwanted living organisms. With ozonated water, a gas is embedded into the water containing 2 extra oxygen atoms for a brief period of time. This makes ozonated water one of the best antiseptics and a great way to get extra oxygen in our bodies. We can't get enough oxygen into our cells and the benefits are tremendous. From anti-cancer to cell rejuvenation to brain function, an abundance of oxygen entering our cells is required for optimal health. A machine is used to pump the extra oxygen into the water, air or oil. The machines are moderately priced and can be used on every glass we drink. The only drawback with ozonated water is it kills the good gut bacteria along with all the other living organisms within us. Probiotics or eating fermented foods may be required to keep the digestive system functioning properly.

Alkaline and Kangen water are both beneficial to good health. These waters can help maintain our alkalinity levels in our blood, and eventually our cells, at a reasonable low pH level. Some of the health benefits of achieving alkalinity throughout our bodies are a reduction of cancer, heart disease, diabetes, and osteoporosis. One drawback is if our body becomes too alkaline, we can expect painful joints and morning stiffness. This condition usually goes away soon after we awake. Creating an alkaline body allows oxygen to be absorbed into our cells more readily.

When we drink water, it automatically goes into an acid environment in our stomachs. This basically nullifies the purpose of alkaline water by diluting our stomach acid to create a difficult environment for our food to be digested. This author believes food should be the best vehicle to achieve alkalinity. Although quality water can help, food can achieve the results faster and more thoroughly than alkaline water alone. If alkaline or Kangen water is consumed, it is advisable to drink this water an hour before meals to allow for gastric emptying to occur. For best results, no liquids should be consumed during meals to allow our stomach the best opportunity to digest its contents.

Water stores are an excellent source for standard water. Standard drinking water has a pH balance very close to neutral, which means it is neither alkaline nor acidic. I have found the purest water comes from the water stores high-quality filters. The aquarium shops can use this untreated water directly into their fish tanks. This water is normally clean and toxin free. Many of these stores now carry alkaline water, along with the standard drinking water.

Home filtration units vary considerably based on design and price. Some units can rival some of the water store waters and some can be slightly better than tap water. The multiple filter systems appear to have the best tasting of water. This author has been impressed with the quality of water from these units. The healthiest way to transport water is in glass. Since glass is natural, no chemicals or residue are leached into the water. If possible, buy glass containers for all your food storage. Ceramic can also be good, however, some manufacturers use a lead based glaze on some of their cookware. As brought up earlier in this book, I was previously an engineer dealing with many toxic materials. My observation recommends all plastics should be avoided. Just our shoes alone is too much exposure to these toxic chemicals. To avoid plastic is unavoidable at this point. Almost everything we purchase is made of plastic. Plastics will leach toxic petroleum-based chemicals into our bodies. These chemicals have created many health issues through prolonged exposure.

As an engineer, I recommend avoiding metal containers, unless made of copper. Aluminum is extremely harmful and has been linked to several mental degenerative illnesses such as Alzheimer's disease. All aluminum cookware should be avoided.

This author is very leery regarding the use of stainless steel. As an engineer working on medical-related products, one of my clients posed a question regarding the toxicity of stainless steel due to the chromium content in this metal. At this time, the European Union was trying to eliminate heavy metals in most of all products. The use of chromium is one of the banned metals which can cause health issues ranging from cancer to mental illness. Since stainless steel has been used for over 100 years in the food and medical industries, I had the curiosity of asking this question to this governing body. I was told to cease all actions and I was threatened to never pursue this topic again. It was a very stern warning that sounded as if something could happen to my personal being. Needless to say, since this encounter, I have regarded stainless steel as a toxic metal ever since.

CHAPTER 6:
How Do I Start?

IS IT TIME TO start your transformation into becoming a healthy person? By now, you should have acquired some knowledge and tools to start this process. If you paid attention, you should know the difference between good and bad food. I hope the human nature and encouragement chapters helped you build your desire for self-improvement. Any type of motivation you may have received is greatly appreciated by this author. Your journey starts now. Not tomorrow or the next day, it starts now. Procrastination is not an option. The graveyard is full of people who procrastinate. If you want to put this health thing off for later, I suggest finding a nice plot at your local cemetery. Unfortunately, with today's horrible food supply, this is where most people will end up, before their time. This reality is sad but true.

The beginning of any new adventure is difficult. Complacency and laziness are the two worst aspects of human nature in regard to change. The first step is always the hardest one to take. This diet is not the most horrible thing you will ever experience. It is only food. Food gives us life. Without food, we would perish rather quickly. Please realize this fact. Your taste buds may hate you for awhile. Your brain may hate you as well, but your body will take over and change the way you think. Your taste buds will begin to enjoy other varieties of food. It's like being a picky eater as a kid. After being forced by your parents to try new foods, your tastes and thinking began to change. Your subconscious took over and certain foods started to taste good. Your body knows what it needs if you listen to it. These dietary changes will become normal and your body will accept these new foods.

Start this diet with an open mind and give it a chance. Just remember, the hatred your taste buds and brain may experience is just temporary. The rest of your body will take over and make this happen. Like explained in a previous chapter, the first six weeks will determine your success or failure. Can you give this diet a chance for six weeks?

This diet is not designed to be a race of any kind. If it were a race it would by a triathlon, long and steady, with no finish line or ending. Since it isn't a race, you will need to start it slowly. Getting used to this diet will allow you a better chance to succeed. Let your body become acclimated to these changes. You may want to start with breakfast at first.

Instead of having Lucky Charms and whole milk for breakfast, you might have a couple of free range eggs with spinach and fried in coconut oil. One of my favorite breakfasts is nopales (cactus), onion, crushed tomato and scrambled eggs, topped with a small avocado. This meal gives your body a balance of protein, complex carbohydrates, and fat. More importantly, it gives you nutrients. This breakfast is loaded with almost every important nutrient for great health. The nutritional properties associated with this meal is outstanding. At around 450 calories, this meal will give your body the nutrients and calories needed to last until lunch, without experiencing hunger. The cactus is a great substitute for meat and it allows your body to utilize carbs more efficiently. The anti-aging and anti-inflammatory properties associated with cactus are extraordinary and beyond anything found on Earth. Remember, your body only wants nutrients, not calories. The calories are on your thigh, butt, and stomach in the form of fat. With this type of breakfast, you will become dependent on your own body fat for energy, instead of the simple carbs from the milk and the Lucky Charms.

By changing one meal at a time, this allows your body to become acclimated to your new diet. Continue with your regular diet for the next week or so, except for the one meal approved by The Infinity Diet.

After this first week, begin to change your snacking habits. Nuts, berries, fruits and vegetables are snacks that should be eaten in between meals before hunger sets in. Nuts are high in calories, but fantastic in good fats and nutrients. An ounce of nuts are fine for a snack, but a bag of nuts are not recommended due to the high-calorie content. The key to long-term success is to never get hungry. Hunger starts a chain of events, which are detrimental to the success of any diet.

Back in our caveman days, food was scarce during the winter month. Our bodies had to adapt to these lean times by producing a stress hormone called cortisol. Since fat contains more calories than protein (9 calories per gram for fat compared to 4 calories per gram for protein), cortisol is dispatched to converts our muscle into fat. This process also halts our metabolism, because our body doesn't have the fuel in our digestive system to keep us energetic. Since it takes 50 calories per pound per day to maintain muscle but only 8 calories per pound to maintain fat, the long-term side effect of this process can cause weight gain when we're able to eat. This process happens quite frequently to people who only eat one meal a day. These individuals are usually overweight and walk around like sloths. The way to combat this problem is to eat low calorie, nutritious foods all day long.

Snacks are critical to succeed on any diet. A steady stream of calories is ideal to combat hunger and maintain your energy. A couple of carrots and a celery stick is an ideal snack. This small 15 calorie burst will curb your appetite until your next meal. Again, your body craves nutrients, not calories.

Being sensible with your snacks is the key. A candy bar in the junk machine is not a snack. It's a treat. My solution was to cut up a bag of veggies every couple of days, so when I felt the slightest twinge of hunger, I can grab a couple pieces to curb my appetite. If you are on an exercise program, a hard-boiled egg or an ounce of nuts may be a better snack. These foods will help combat muscle loss caused by a protein deficiency. The exercise program will increase your metabolism significantly, so these added calories will not matter. Eggs and nuts are very nutrient rich foods.

By the third week, change another meal in your diet. This is where meal prepping becomes very important. Since we can't guarantee the integrity of most prepared foods, bringing your own lunch to work is the best solution. A salad or leftover spaghetti squash in marinara sauce could be a wonderful lunch. If your busy schedule forces you to purchase a lunch, Chipotle is an acceptable choice, since they advertise an all organic menu. The only avoidable items on their menu are rice, chips, tofu, cheese and sour cream. Flame Broiler, Yoshinoya, and Subway all have items approved by The Infinity Diet, however, these establishments do not advertise organic foods. The foods to avoid on their menus are rice, bread, and cheese. A lettuce wrapped hamburger or lettuce wrapped grilled chicken sandwich is also acceptable it a pinch. However, these ingredients may be suspect.

By the fourth week, everything you eat should meet the criteria of The Infinity Diet. Dinner is the most difficult to control if you have a family. The temptations created by your friends or family can make you give in to eat poorly. My favorite solution is to take charge and use a little psychology to stick to your diet. When your friends or family want to go out for dinner, be strong and make a point to have everyone eat healthy. Choose a restaurant with healthy choices on their menu and don't be swayed by peer pressure. If you end up at a pizza parlor for a birthday party, eat a salad. Chinese food restaurants usually offer an abundance of foods that meet The Infinity Diet criteria. If you absolutely have no choice but to eat badly, make sure it is one of your cheat meals. Later in this book, I will explain how cheating on your diet is very beneficial to achieve success. Being strict all the time makes us less human. Everyone needs to let loose a little.

Since dinner is so close to bedtime, this is the most critical meal of the day. We could have a negative calorie diet the whole day and still gain fat overnight if we're not careful. When we sleep, our body changes drastically. Our metabolism actually increases during our rest time. To recover from the damage we inflict upon ourselves on a daily basis, we must sleep at least 7 hours per night. During our rest time, protein and nutrients are required for full recovery. If we eat a carb-laden dinner before bed, these carbs will not be utilized correctly and they will turn directly into fat. Pasta, bread, dairy, and rice should be avoided for dinner. These foods are easily turned into sugar. A vegetable and meat meal is much more advisable. Many of us have eaten a spaghetti dinner with garlic bread and ice cream for dessert. I know it tastes good, but the weight gain associated with this meal is tremendous due to the overabundance of carbohydrates. This meal sitting in our digestive system overnight can cause health issues and weight gain.

Late night snacks are acceptable on The Infinity Diet. If you had eaten a sensible dinner and you feel a little hungry before bed, please eat something with protein. An ounce of nuts or a piece of chicken can curb your appetite and provide needed protein for recovery.

Protein does not turn into fat while we sleep, carbs do. If we consume too much protein before bed, our kidneys will eliminate the leftover protein through our urine in the morning. Remember, hunger produces cortisol and so does the lack of sleep. Make sure you eat enough protein at night and get plenty of sleep for full recovery.

By the fifth week, your body should be fully acclimated to your new diet. You will start to feel healthier, but not very energetic. The energy levels usually increase around the seventh week. By this time, your body will be in full-fat burning mode. However, your body's desire to burn sugar will still be in effect. At this point, your body hasn't quite realized that fat and complex carbs will be its new energy source.

You may notice your body fat softening. This means the fat cells are releasing some of their toxins, therefore allowing the correct nutrients to start the flushing process. It's possible to experience some minor signs of Herxheimer Syndrome, explained earlier. You will also notice your clothes starting to fit a little looser. The mirror and your clothes sizes should be your visible judge, not the scale. Your friends and family may start to notice your physical changes. When you begin to hear kind words being said about your appearance, this is when your brain fully gives in and accepts this new lifestyle change. The power of the brain is grossly under appreciated.

To avoid resuming your old lifestyle, try to make subtle changes to your family's diet. As much as you want to force feed this diet onto your loved ones, they have to come to their own realization. For your sake and their health, let's hope awareness comes sooner than later. Usually one of your kids or spouse will join you on this new adventure soon after you begin. This will add some fun to your journey. When it comes to people's health, being a role model is the best path to take. Inspire their desire to change.

CHAPTER 7:
I Can Eat What!!!!

A FAMOUS GREEK PHYSICIAN named Hippocrates once said, "Let food be thy medicine and medicine be thy food". This guy knew what he was talking about 2,300 years ago. If we follow his principals, we will stay healthy. If we don't, guess what, we get illness and death. You pick!!! All our medicine once came from nature. Humans have found a way to artificially take these compounds to recreate chemical versions for the sake of profits. Are these chemicals the same as the natural sources? The answer is not even close. Whatever your belief system may be, either nature or god created everything we need to flourish on the planet. Humankind's quest for wealth has taken this natural medical system and essentially killed it through the media and legislation.

Lies and corruption have taken precedence over natural health. The saddest part is most people are gullible and ignorant. They believe what they hear. I think it's time to end all this corruption. This book should be an awakening. People need to go back to the basics and use food to prevent all these man-made diseases created by our capitalistic society. Let the ignorant remain unhealthy and let the rest of us attend their funerals.

Can you imagine going to the doctor and your doctor prescribed dandelion root tea to treat your liver condition? I would go to my neighbor's yard and pull some weeds. My neighbor would be happy and so would my liver. This is the type of medicine the eastern world uses to treat illnesses.

Almost every illness has a natural remedy to treat or cure the problem we may be experiencing. For instance, men with low testosterone should avoid beer and soy products and consume more cabbage. Resistant training is also one of the best natural testosterone boosters. Do you think your doctor knows this bit of natural medicine? Probably not. Your doctor will look into his iPad like a crystal ball and sees that AndroGel is the most highly prescribed medicine for this condition. Do you think he'll prescribe cabbage and lifting weights instead? Probably not, since Androgel is profitable and cabbage is not. AndroGel is a dangerous steroid which can cause damage to your liver, kidneys and reproductive organs along with increasing your chances of acquiring prostate cancer. Cabbage is a vegetable full of vitamins and minerals. Which one would you take? I knew it, the AndroGel. That's because we're all brainwashed into thinking our doctors are acting in our best interest. Actually, your doctor was probably thinking about his best interest, not yours. When he wrote the prescription, your doctor was actually planning his free trip to Las Vegas paid by Big Pharma.

The Infinity Diet is very simple and easy to follow. The main two food groups to eliminate or severely restrict are grains and cow-based dairy. Neither of these groups provides enough long-term value for our health or longevity. Grains are the cheapest way to feed the masses and cow-based dairy is nothing more than dead bacteria, sugar, protein, and water. Let's break down these avoidable foods to see what they truly provide nutritionally.

Grains consist of wheat, oats, barley, rice, corn, rye and various other products. The Infinity Diet restricts their use because all grains are processed into simple sugar in our digestive system. Simple sugars have been linked to obesity, heart disease, fatty liver disease and especially cancer. Most grains are naturally high in minerals, yet low in vitamins. Almost all the vitamins added to grain come from artificial sources. The one nutrient which needs to be avoided is fortified iron, found in all processed wheat. This nutrient has been linked to arterial sclerosis when combined with animal protein and calcium. The hardening of the arteries is the leading cause of strokes and heart attacks. 50% of all victims show little signs of heart issues before their fatal or near fatal event. Calcium becomes solidified in our circulatory system when these three ingredients are combined. When a piece of razor sharp calcium breaks away and punctures the circulatory wall, a blood clot can form. It is cholesterol's job to patch up the puncture to prevent a clot. However, if the puncture is too large and cholesterol isn't able to contain the clot, a stroke or heart attack will occur. These facts make our breakfast cereal and milk a deadly combination.

Since sugar is the primary fuel for cancer, the use of grains should be restricted. Cancer can't survive without sugar and it will starve to death. If we limit our grains and other sugars, cancer won't have the fuel to flourish, thus eliminating the chances of contracting this deadly disease. This vital clue is part of the cure for cancer. Has a doctor ever talked to you about this fact? I doubt it since doctors only receive 2 days of nutrition lessons in their 8 years of school. A broken system creates broken patients.

Grains are dead foods and are acidic by nature, while live foods are very alkaline and nutritious. Since cancer thrives in an acid environment, eliminating acidic foods will decrease your chances of contracting this disease when combined with a non-sugar diet. This is the 2nd leading clue for the cure for cancer. Overall, the negative associated with grain consumption outweighs the benefit by a large margin.

Today's wheat poses several health concerns to our population. Not only is wheat fortified with iron, wheat also has been linked to serious digestive issues mentioned in chapter 5. The final concern associated with wheat is its use in processed baked goods. Yeast is a living organism used to make bread and cakes rise. If yeast is not used, our baked goods would be hard and flat, similar to a thick tortilla. Recent studies have shown that yeast may play a significant role in the production of cancer cells, along with dairy products. The center of every cancer cell is a living microbe. These microbes seem to come from foods with high levels of fungus and bacteria. The yeast in these products dies during the baking process but reemerges during cooling. If we eat any bread or pastries, be aware of the pitfalls associated with yeast. In chapter 15, I will explain how to eliminate this threat from living microbes.

Corn poses several different problems to our health. Unfortunately, all the issues associated with corn are man-made. Organic corn as a vegetable is approved by The Infinity Diet, however other corn products are banned. As explained earlier, corn is a GMO product. Since GMO corn can be made into inexpensive oil, corn syrup and used as feed for most of our meat sources, this makes corn one of the main contributors to poor health. Corn oil is very high in Omega 6's, which should be limited, as explained earlier. Although a good source of Vitamin E, this out of balance use of Omega 6's compared to Omega 3's makes corn oil undesirable. The biggest issue regarding corn is the use of chemicals to genetically modify this plant. The GMO issue remains the single most destructive element in today's food supply. The widespread use of GMO corn and soybeans is creating severe health issues in today's society.

High fructose corn syrup has taken over as the sugar of choice by most food manufacturers. This product is inexpensive to produce and very profitable. Is high fructose corn syrup good for us? This author believes this product should be banned for human consumption, period!!! It appears to be the #1 cause of obesity today. When we ingest this garbage, our digestive system doesn't know what to do with it. Since it isn't a natural food, our digestive system passes the buck to the liver for a solution. Our liver is the main factory for all our important body functions. Since our liver can't figure it out either, it stores this crap as fat to be used for a rainy day. As we continue to eat this junk, our bodies keep storing it and it is never utilized as energy. This storing effect is creating fatty liver disease, diabetic issues, and obesity. Therefore, high fructose corn syrup is the main cause of today's childhood obesity and diabetic issues. Most of the junk food children crave is laced with this garbage. Almost every soda, salad dressing, bread, peanut butter, breakfast cereal, and jelly is made with this non-digestible crap.

Many of today's illnesses began when the food industry decided to use corn to feed the animals bred for mass consumption. Since corn was never part of the animal diet in the first place, this corn feed ferments and breeds bacteria in their stomach. Such bacterial illnesses as E-Coli, Salmonella, Listeria, and Botulism are now present in our eggs, pork, beef, and chicken. Milk would have these same issues if it weren't for homogenizing. When we consume any animal based products, please cook the food thoroughly. A temperature of at least 165 degrees should be reached before eating such foods. The heating process will kill the harmful bacteria. As explained earlier, we have to contend with the GMO issues as well. It takes us the consumers to change this system. The population needs to stop buying these tainted products for this industry to take notice.

As discussed earlier, cow-based dairy products should not be consumed by humans. The negatives associated with these products outweigh any of benefit we may experience from their use. Along with the health issues associated with cow dairy, dairy products, such as cheese, tend to add extra pounds to your body. I call it Baby Fat Syndrome. If you have ever observed breastfed babies, they tend to be fatter than babies given formula. I believe breast milk fat is the cause of this condition. The same thing happens to adults who consume dairy products. Our bodies appear to retain dairy fat more readily than other fats. Thus, the overuse of cheese and high fructose corn syrup are two of the main reason why obesity is so prevalent in today's society.

The over-promotion of cheese in almost all our convenience foods has become an epidemic and our population's addiction to cheese is out of control. When will this overuse slow down? Only when the majority of the citizens reduce their consumption will this epidemic cease. Remember, most toxins are stored in fat cells. Therefore, cheese is nothing more than high calorie, aged fat toxins. On our bodies, this is the hard body fat we feel around our midsection. If health and longevity are a concern, dairy products should be eliminated or greatly reduced. Also, dairy bacteria is very similar to the yeast found in bread and baked goods explained earlier in this chapter. The same types of illnesses can be associated with the use of these two highly microbial products.

There is one dairy product that all people should eat on a daily basis. This food is a paste, similar to mayonnaise, made from either organic cottage cheese, goat or sheep kefir and freshly ground flax seeds along with flax seed oil. Dr. Johanna Budwig was a German biochemistry expert in the use of fats, who made this incredible discovery. She found that by combining these ingredients into a paste at a ratio of 2 part dairy to 1 part flax seed oil with a tablespoon of freshly ground flax seeds, this paste became water soluble. This meant that our cells could ingest this paste like water. She found that highly unsaturated fat combined with a sulfur based protein could reenergize our cells at an incredible rate. As we age, our cells lose their electrical charge. This paste restores our electrical charge back to our teenage years and decreases the time required to reproduce new cells. By consuming this paste along with a vegetable based diet, many illnesses such as cancer, diabetes, eczema, psoriasis, arthritis, Alzheimer's disease, Parkinson's disease, dementia, hormonal issues and heart disease can be stopped or cured with a success rate of between 80-93%. This incredible breakthrough was suppressed by the medical establishment because well people are less profitable than sick people. Just think of the millions of people who could have been cured by this wonderful paste. They were cured in Germany, but this information was never made available to the general public in the United States. I believe this formula is the greatest discovery in medical history. The anti-aging properties alone are incredible. This formula could bankrupt our Social Security system by itself. For this paste to work correctly, the consumption of any other processed fats can't be eaten for 3 hours after its initial use. The consumption of these fats will nullify its healing properties. This paste can be blended with berries, nuts, and honey for a wonderful sweet dip or combined with cayenne pepper or turmeric for a spicy mixture. I like to eat this paste as a dip for my vegetables. This is the only dairy product approved by The Infinity Diet and rightfully so. This paragraph is worth more than all your health care costs combined if you use this invaluable formula. Under The Infinity Diet, the consumption of meat is allowed a couple times a week. As explained in the previous chapter, meat has many pitfalls but is required for proper cell rejuvenation. Although amino acids can be found in other foods and supplements, these animal-based proteins convert to higher quality amino acids for muscle and cell health. Studies have shown the human body needs about 4 ounces of meat, twice a week for proper muscle rejuvenation. Remember, your heart is also a muscle. By having a constant supply of amino acids in our digestive system, the other proteins in our foods can be better utilized. Every living organism needs protein to sustain life, but only meat and soybeans have all the required amino acids. Since meat takes around 3 days to digest, these amino acids are always available in our digestive tract. NASA uses this blueprint to locate for life on other planets.

Consuming a little meat is great for our muscles and cells, however eating too much will halt our metabolism. Since meat is hard to digest, your body slows to a crawl in order to process this food. Have you ever watched a nature program with lions and tigers? If you have, these huge cats will normally eat 20 lbs of a deer or antelope in one sitting. Afterward, the cat will climb a tree and sleep for the next two weeks while this meat is digesting. The same thing happens to us. Remember reading this paragraph the next time you overindulge on meat. What do you want to do after that meal? That's right, you want to sleep. Your body needs all its energy for digestion, just like the cat on the television. Studies have shown that when your metabolism is high, the aging process slows. This is one reason why thin people tend to live a lot longer than overweight people. Their motor is running at a high rate of speed, while the overweight person has trouble getting out of their own way. The plan is to eat small quantities of meat to keep our muscles and cells healthy, but not enough to slow down our metabolism. Try to eat extremely lean meat, since most toxins are stored in the fat. All vegetables are allowed on The Infinity Diet, except for soybeans. As previously explained, soy products shut down our thyroid function, increase our human growth hormone and estrogen levels. The majority of soybeans are also grown from GMO seeds. Although increased growth hormone and high estrogen levels can benefit some individuals, destroying our thyroid function and having GMO induced digestive issues will outweigh any good associated with this plant, especially for men.

The health benefits associated with eating vegetables is tremendous. From being alkaline and high in oxygen to supplying most of all key nutrients, vegetables are the best food for longevity and weight control. All vegetables range from neutral pH to highly alkaline. Most infectious illnesses live in an acid environment. Therefore, eating vegetables will prevent many diseases.

Vegetables are like oxygen factories. They breathe in carbon dioxide and exhale oxygen, while animals breathe oxygen and exhale carbon dioxide. This oxygen enters our digestive system and reenergizes our cells. Each cell can't replicate without the presence of oxygen. This is the main factor why some people remain healthy, while others become sick. We want our cells to rejuvenate as quickly as possible to keep us young and vibrant throughout our lives. People with stagnant cells, caused by the lack of oxygen, tend to develop many debilitating illnesses. The combination of exercise and vegetables will increase your lifespan considerably. As explained throughout this book, ozonated water, exercise, vegetables and the Budwig Diet hold all the keys to living a high-quality life for many years past the average life expectancy.

Every nutrient imaginable can be found in fruits and vegetables, except for vitamin B12 and vitamin D. The best sources for vitamin B12 are animal-based foods and for vitamin D is the sun. Wheatgrass, for instance, has 98 out of the 102 keys nutrients needed for optimal health. The benefits associated with a vegetable dependant diet are endless. From curing cancer to having beautiful hair, vegetables should be your food of choice for health and longevity. Remember, if it came from the ground, eat it. The only drawbacks related to consuming vegetables are man-made issues. Pesticides and GMO products are what should be avoided. As emphasized in a previous chapter, try to eat either organic or home grown produce. If store bought produce is your only recourse, make sure to soak the vegetables in either ozonated water or vinegar to release many of the pesticides and chemicals. Some of the GMO vegetables listed include zucchini, yellow squash, corn, soybeans, sugar beets, tomatoes, and potatoes. If possible, try to buy the organic versions of these products or eliminate these vegetables from your diet. The only natural concern comes from raw spinach. Spinach should be heated above 135 degrees before consumption. Spinach contains an acid called oxalate, which binds other minerals together to form kidney stones, especially magnesium and calcium.

All fruit is permitted on The Infinity Diet in moderation. Due to the high content of fructose sugar, limiting your fruit intake to a couple of pieces a day is beneficial for proper nutrition. As explained earlier, fruit is essentially the same as vegetables, except for the sugar, which doubles the calories by weight. The best fruit to consume for dieting purposes is berries and citrus. Berries are natural fat burners and citrus can increases your metabolism. Grapefruit is also wonderful for your heart. If you have ever noticed, many heart medications suggest not eating grapefruit while taking this medicine. The reason is grapefruit is also a wonderful heart medicine. It essentially doubles the dosage of whatever medication your doctor has prescribed for your condition. Shouldn't doctors prescribe grapefruit for a treatment instead? The pharmaceutical companies wouldn't like that very much; however, your body would love it. Apples also have anti-cancer properties and are wonderful at fighting off free radicals. Free radicals are waste products caused by a chemical reaction in our cells. These waste products are accumulated and tend to attack our healthy cells. Many illnesses associated with free radical damage are cancer, Alzheimer's disease, arterial sclerosis, arthritis and many other illnesses. Alcohol, tobacco, aging and prescription medications are some of the causes associated with the formation of free radicals. By eliminating toxins from our air, water, food and bad habits, we can hold the free radicals at bay with proper nutrition. Anti-oxidants are the best free radical fighters. Several different fruits are full of antioxidants, especially berries and citrus.

Pineapples are wonderful at breaking down proteins. This fruit contains an enzyme called bromelain which makes our bodies utilize the proteins more efficiently. Bromelain can also help produce a better insulin response for diabetics. Athletes can benefit by eating pineapples to decrease their recovery time.

A few varieties of apples, tomatoes and especially papaya are now GMO foods. Again, try to find organic sources for these particular foods to ensure proper health. This is extremely disturbing since papaya is one of the best probiotic foods known, along with ginger root. Probiotics have essential enzymes and bacteria needed to break down our foods during digestion.

Nuts and seeds are wonderful sources of good fats, nutrients, fiber, and protein. All types of nuts and seeds should be consumed on The Infinity Diet. The only drawback regarding seeds and nuts is they are very calories dense. Therefore, if you choose to eat nuts and seeds, limit yourself to 2 ounces per day. Each variety has their own unique health benefit associated with their consumption. For instance, Brazil nuts are extremely high in selenium. Selenium is one of the best cancer fighters known to humankind. This mineral can shut off the mutation of cancer cells. Only three Brazil nuts a day can give you this wonderful miracle. Another fantastic nut is the almond. Almonds are extremely high in an amino acid called L-Arginine. In 1998, 3 Norwegian doctors won the Nobel Prize for medicine for their research on the incredible amino acid. The results of their study showed that L-Arginine can remove all the plaque in our circulatory system, normalize the cholesterol levels in our blood and remove some of the accumulated blood sugar as a result of diabetes. In other words, it was determined L-Arginine can rid humanity of three of the four main reasons why people die, heart attack, stroke, and diabetes. Do you think your doctor will prescribe almonds as a treatment for your heart disease or diabetes? I could only hope so in the near future. By ridding our blood stream of these undesired entities, our blood can flow smoother and faster. Faster blood flow has been associated with increased metabolism, which means, almond will make you lose weight, in spite their calories. I suggest eating a variety of nuts and seeds to reap all the benefits associated with these wonderful creations.

Peanuts come from the legume family and are not considered a nut. Though similar to nuts, peanuts are closer to the nutritional values of their cousins, the bean. Beans are also approved for consumption on The Infinity Diet. Legumes are wonderful sources of protein, iron, potassium, phosphorus, magnesium, calcium and fiber. Since legumes are high in protein and low in sugar, beans should be consumed by diabetics, especially white beans. White beans tend to regulate the blood sugar by increasing the insulin response. Freshly made beans are more nutritious than the canned variety due to the added salt content.

There are a couple drawbacks regarding the use of legume in our diets. Soybeans and other soy products come from the legume family and should be avoided at all costs for various reasons explained earlier in this chapter. Legumes need to be thoroughly cooked before consumption because legumes are actually poisonous in their raw form. The heating process eliminates the poison and allows us to eat these products without any side effects. Legumes also contain live bacteria. These bacteria, along with yeast and dairy products, have been shown to form the microbe nucleus associated with many different cancers. This information should not be of any significance to you since your body's immune system will be working at such a high level. Unhealthy people should be concerned with their immune system not working up to its capacity.

As an overview, grains, and dairy should be limited, if not avoided in this diet. Lean meats should be limited to a couple serving a week to allow their amino acids to help break down other dietary proteins. Vegetables should be consumed as the staple food for this diet. The health benefits of consuming vegetables are tremendous for both weight maintenance and longevity. Fruit should be limited to a couple of pieces a day, due to its high fructose sugar content. Nuts and seeds should be limited to a couple ounces per day, due to the high-calorie content associated with these foods. Legumes can be consumed anytime due to their high protein content and nutritional value.

Now you should have enough tools to start your journey to health and prosperity. I hope you allowed this information to sink in because your quality of life will depend on it. Get ready, get set, go!!! Now start the slowest race of your life today!!!

CHAPTER 8:
So What Does Exercise Have To Do With Diet!!!!

IN CHAPTER 3, I EXPLAINED to achieve great health, it requires 90% diet and 10% exercise. However, good health can be achieved by diet alone. By adding exercise to your diet, you will reap tremendous benefits for the rest of your life. I would take great health over good health any day. Many health issues can be prevented if exercise is added as the icing on your cake to longevity. Such conditions as bone and muscle loss can be prevented as we age. When we add maintaining our flexibility and balance into our cake mixture, our quality of life will increase substantially. Isn't this the premise of the book? Why should we suffer through illness all our lives? I personally would rather not use a cane or allow anyone to wipe my butt as I age. Being self-sufficient throughout our lives will bring us happiness and joy. Others who don't respect their bodies will experience pain and suffering. Since you decided to buy this book, I know which path you chose. Now it's time to go back to our science lesson once again.

A suppressed 6-month study on how resistance training can combat the aging process was performed in 2007. This study consisted of 26 older physically active volunteers with the average age of 68 and 25 younger relatively inactivity volunteers with an average age of 24. All the subjects had muscle and DNA samples extracted from their bodies prior to the study.

What the researchers discovered was of the 30,000 or so genes in the human body, roughly 29,400 of the genes do not change as we age. Only 596 genes actually degrade as we get older. A known fact is around the age of 40, humans start to lose their muscle mass because of aging and poor living habits. Science has shown this is caused by oxidative stress and a lack of anti-oxidants being consumed to prevent this condition called sarcopenia. This study was performed to see if the older subjects could actually halt their muscle loss through resistance training. The researchers had the older subjects start a full body weight training program, which consisted of workouts twice a week for six months. Initially, the older subjects were 59% weaker than the younger subjects. After the 6 month study, the older subjects were only 38% weaker than the younger subjects. Therefore, the older subjects became considerably stronger.

At the conclusion of the study, the researchers again took muscle and DNA samples from 14 of the 26 older subjects for testing. What they found was astonishing, Out of the 596 genes identified by the aging process, 417 of these genes remained unchanged and the other 179 actually showed considerable signs of regression. The researchers knew they found the fountain of youth. If people consistently worked their muscles after the age of 40, the aging process would not progress.

These researchers took their findings to be published, but the media squashed their efforts. The report was never published or sent out through any media channels. What will healthy old people do to our society, except kill off medical insurance and Social Security? It appears the powers above want the elderly sick and dying for profitability purposes. Profitability over humanity is the theme we have to tolerate within today's society. I feel it's time for us to do our own squashing. Let's burden society with a bunch of productive old people because this is our life. We are not cash cows that can be slaughtered after our money runs out. I understand a need for population control in today's society, but if we go back 150 years, people were self-sustaining. We can plant our own food and raise our own animals again. Laws and regulations are now set to prohibit this natural lifestyle. I understand we need laws to control wayward activities, but when it comes to life, the regulations should be left to the more important issues. Try to get your neighbors involved by starting an urban garden and sustain your own healthy style of living. If everyone decided to make these changes; the elderly would not be a burden to the younger generations.

When it comes to exercise, science says slow resistance interval training, balance and stretching are the best forms of exercise for the human body. Slow resistance interval training maintains your muscle function without destroying your bones and joints. Balance and stretching exercises, such as yoga, are critical to maintaining a high quality of life. As we age, we tend to lose these physical abilities. The saying "Use it, don't lose it" couldn't be more correct. As children, we might have wrestled our friends and walked on railroad tracks. As adults, our physical activity gradually decreases due to several factors, such as laziness, busy schedules, injuries, and complacency. If we maintain an active lifestyle like children, these abilities will never be lost. The main premise of physical exercise is JUST MOVE YOUR BODY. With childhood obesity and the video era upon us, humankind may face a tremendous epidemic of medical issues in the very near future.

With most physical activity, our body and mind will reap the benefit. There are a few exceptions. Some exercise programs go past our own physical limitations. In the sake of competition, these activities have validity. However, for the average person, some of these programs appear to create tremendous health on the outside but destroy our bodies from the inside. Do you think a 60-year-old housewife should take up power lifting? I could see a 25-year-old mom taking up this activity for the sake of competition. Will this mom have physical damage as a result of her training? The answer is probably yes. She will experience degenerative hips and knees and experience shoulder issues as she ages. Our competitive nature can drive us to perform such activities with reckless abandon. This type of exercise is good for our mental health and increases the "feel goods" we experience. Many chemicals are released through our glands to give us that high many of us long for. Ultimately, is this exercise good for her? Her answer today is yes, but tomorrow her answer may change. My personal experience as a high fly basketball player in my teens and 20's told me I should've considered a different sport. I have degenerative joints all over my body and experience chronic pain on a daily basis. I have many physical limitations today, due to this competitive sport. My basketball life was cut short due to the injuries I incurred. Today, I can only wish for a pain-free quality of life. It's too late for me now. I hope this advice will help you on your journey to long lasting health and a pain-free existence.

When it comes to muscle health, slow resistance interval training appears to be the best form of exercise for all ages. Slow resistance required weights or some type of training apparatus which puts a strain on our muscles. By doing resistance training in a slow, methodical manner with relatively light weight, the muscles are utilized to the fullest, without the possibility of bone or joint damage. Over time, the muscles will strengthen and reverse degenerative muscle loss associated with aging. This type of training will also strengthen the joints and bones to relieve the effects of osteoporosis and arthritis if we adhere to the dietary restraints of The Infinity Diet. If you start this program in your early years, you will experience life with strength and ease. Everyday life is easier for a fit person, compared to an unfit person. Just image how much easier it would be to mop the floor or do laundry if your body was working to its fullest. Wouldn't be nice to be able to play catch with your kids or ride a bike at the beach with the family? Your children will remember all these life-changing experiences you shared with them as they get older. Many parents today are so unhealthy and can only wish to experience these wonderful moments with their children. Resistance training can help you regain your quality of life once again or allow you to experience it for the first time.

The premise to this type of training is to tax the muscles to the point of failure and rest 30 seconds to 1 minute between exercises. Muscle damage is needed to strengthen and rebuild the muscles in this type of training. Many people just go through the motions and stop at a certain number of repetitions. This type of training is only teasing the muscles and little benefit is experienced. The premise is to push yourself until your muscles fail. There is no magic number to achieve. When your brain tells you to stop, rest for 30 sec to 1 minute for recovery and repeat the exercise again. Keep repeating this exercise until your muscles fail completely. After muscle failure is achieved, go to another exercise and repeat the same process in a different muscle group. This creates interval training, which is wonderful for your heart. While exercising, you will reach an acceptable heart rate. As you rest in between sets, your heart rate will decrease slightly, resulting in the desired effect most researchers say is the key to achieving a healthy heart.

By exercising with slow resistance, the explosive muscles are worked and their complimentary muscles are taxed at the same time. With this type of training, you can basically double the efficiency of your workouts and limit the abuse to your bones and joints created by this slow and deliberate motion. This type of training is used with lighter weights because there is no momentum used to move the weight. The weight is only moved by your strength. Therefore, your muscles will be fully engaged during the extent of each exercise, making this form of training extremely effective. To add a twist to your training, at some point during the set, hold the weight in a tense position for five seconds and explode afterward. This is called a static. Statics tax the muscles tremendously and increase the strength of the muscle beyond the normal exercise. With little tension on the bones and joints, this movement is very beneficial to the success of this type of training.

Rest plays an important role in slow resistant interval training. Since we are taxing our muscles to failure, the muscles need time to heal. If we refuse to allow enough time for repair, we will keep stripping our bodies of critical muscle mass. Over time, the body will become weaker physically and this can cause a compromised immune system. There is only so much healing a human body can do. As we age, the healing process slows considerably. However, science has shown several natural ways to accelerate the healing process. One way is to take anti-oxidant supplements or eat foods rich in anti-oxidants. Vitamin A, C, E, zinc, and selenium are the key anti-oxidant to increase the healing process. Free radicals also love damaged muscle and are the major cause of muscle soreness. If we combat the free radicals with anti-oxidants, the soreness will be greatly reduced and the healing process will accelerate tremendously. The general rule of thumb of healing for people experiencing muscle failure is one day of rest for every 10 years of age. Otherwise, a person 30 years of age should rest the failed muscle group for 3 days, while a 50-year-old should rest 5 days. If you follow this rule, your muscles should be fully recovered by the time your next session begins using the same muscle group. If any soreness still exists, wait until the soreness subsides. There is no use stripping damaged muscles away like explained earlier. Recovery is the key to success. Resist the human tendency to go back to soon. Remember, there are many different muscle groups you can work instead. Work smarter, not harder. Your body will respond better with a little consideration.

As we age, balance and flexibility are extremely important to longevity. Many of the injuries which occur in our twilight years are caused by losing these certain essential abilities. To maintain our functionality, I suggest yoga. Not only is yoga wonderful at connecting our minds to our body, yoga remains the greatest form of exercise to reintroduce these lost abilities. This non-evasive program will strengthen the joints, stretch your muscles and activate your abdominal core, which many of us have lost over the years. Yoga is great for all ages and levels of ability.

Although intensive cardio has many health benefits associated with our heart and increasing the oxygen levels in our cells, this form of exercise causes premature aging. If we choose to do any sort of cardio work, keep the workout below 20 minutes. True cardio is not needed for longevity. By using the slow resistant interval training method, your heart rate will remain high enough to reap the same benefits as cardio.

People use three forms of energy while they exercise. Each

form is dependent on your choice of activity. The first energy source is known as anaerobic, which means without oxygen. This energy is used while doing such activities as sprinting or weight training. This fuel source is needed for explosive exercises which last up to two minutes in length. The anaerobic energy source comes from stored sugar which resides in our muscle tissue. When the sugar is depleted from our muscles, lactate becomes our next energy source. Lactate is the leftover sugar in our muscles combining with oxygen to create a chemical called ATP or adenosine triphosphate. When ATP is burned in our muscles, it creates lactic acid. Lactic acid causes temporary muscle fatigue and soreness. Our ATP supply can last everywhere from 2 to 20 minutes before we begin to use our final energy source, which is fat. When fat becomes our last fuel source, our body starts to shut down. The body tends to store fat for lean times, like hunger. If we start to use fat as our primary fuel source, our metabolism grinds to a halt and the stress hormone cortisol decided to rear its ugly head. Cortisol is used to preserve our fat storage through the use of our lean muscle. This is the reason prolonged cardio activities accelerates the aging process. The general rule is if you want to eat and sleep after exercising, you have over trained. While we sleep, our body wants to use the food to replenish the fat we had lost during your workout. Under these circumstances, our body will become fatter every time we over train.

After we exercise, our bodies need to replenish the fuels and nutrients we lose during our workout. Studies have shown the best post workout formula for recovery is eating a combination of fast digesting protein and carbs. While most exercise enthusiasts like to use whey as their post workout protein source, whey is actually a leftover dairy product from the cheese industry. This junk used be thrown away until it was analyzed and found to be high in protein. I believe it still belongs in the trash. This heavily microbial waste product has been linked to a severely increased risk of cancer. This garbage in a tub is usually laden with a bunch of chemicals, which cause a heavy burden on the liver. The best part of whey protein is it's very profitable. It doesn't get any better for profitability than going from the trash to our mouth. I believe whey protein is the ultimate product for our capitalistic society. Most of these whey protein products contain aspartic acid as a testosterone booster. Although this acid does increase your hormone levels, it also is one of the leading causes of impotence in males.

Research has shown the best meal for recovery is breakfast with eggs. Eggs are the fastest digestible source of protein. As soon as your workout is completed, recovery needs to start. Otherwise, cortisol and the free radicals will begin to cause havoc to your body. To prevent this destruction from occurring, an anti-oxidant cocktail is required. The ideal post workout meal should include something with eggs, carrots, broccoli, fruit and nuts. These foods have the all the necessary nutrients required for a wonderful recovery. So how does a broccoli, carrot and egg omelet with fruit and nuts as a dessert sound to you? It sounds kind of good to me.

A 4 to 1 ratio of carbs to protein is the magic number found by researchers for the United States Olympic Team for post workout meals. The best part about this meal is it counts as zero calories. Since your body uses all of its nutrients for immediate recovery and to replenish the lost sugars stored in your muscles, this meal won't add any fat to your body. As explained earlier, your protein requirement will vary based on the amount of lean muscle mass your body possesses. Based on your muscle content, you may have to consume anywhere from 20 to 75 grams of protein to 80 to 300 grams of carbs for your post workout meal to replenish your depleted nutrients.

The strangest part regarding this meal is it becomes your energy source for your next workout. What happens is when the digested proteins turn into amino acids for muscle recovery, the sugar from your meal attaches to the amino acid molecules for a piggy back ride into your muscles. This sugar storage is the energy needed for your next workout session. With a little knowledge, we can achieve the best possible results.

CHAPTER 9:

What is this Alkaline Stuff All About?

WHEN IT COMES TO overall health, there are three main components to staying healthy. The first is to take in plenty of oxygen. This doesn't mean to breathe more. It means to eat more oxygen based foods like fruits and vegetables and to move your body. When we're active, our heart rate increases and our bodies need more oxygen. Living in the concrete jungle of a large city, people are naturally oxygen deleted. As time passes, more and more land is covered in concrete and the forests are being cut down. Our big city's oxygen levels have been depleted by as much as 50% in the past 50 years and 35% is the average for most of today's large metropolitan areas. This reduction of oxygen is causing many lung and brain conditions. The increase of greenhouse gasses, such as carbon dioxide, is causing further brain and cell diseases. Therefore, for a long healthy life, a rural climate is much more desirable. Studies have shown the life expectancy of people living in large cities is about 10 years less than those living in a rural setting. It appears living in a healthy environment also translates to living a longer, healthier life.

The second main component is to eliminate simple sugar from your diet. Since the food industry began using sugar in all our foods, the increase of illnesses has also increased by a huge margin. Such illnesses as diabetes, heart disease, obesity, and cancer are all associated with high sugar diets. Today, studies have shown that the average person eats between 150 and 170 lbs of sugar per year. That's about a 1/2 a pound a day!!! If you compared this in historical content, in 1700 the average person ate only 8 pounds per year. In 1800, the average person ate 18 lbs per year and in 1900, the average person increased to 60 lbs per year. The people of today are now eating about 800 calories of sugar per day, while in 1800; people ate 88 calories per day. This is a great indicator of why obesity has become such an epidemic in today's society.

There are also many other illnesses caused by obesity, such as liver and kidney disease. The worst one of all diseases is cancer. The cancer rates in the United States are currently one in every two people will contract this deadly disease sometime during their lifetime. The main source of fuel for cancer is sugar. Do you see a correlation to this increased cancer rate? Studies have shown if cancer patients eliminate their sugar intake, their cancer cannot survive. Has any doctor ever explained this fact to you? Since doctors only receive two days of nutrition in their 8 years of study, I don't think so. I doubt if your doctor even knows this critical bit of information. This book should educate you better than your doctor has probably ever learned about natural health. Although, your doctor can kick your butt on what pills to take, in which he is an expert. Anyway, the law specifies that chemo, radiation, and surgery are the only allowed treatments for cancer. So your doctor can't legally tell you about this information even if he knew it. He would be at risk of prosecution and he couldn't buy his vacation home in Costa Rica from jail.

The last component is acidity. Our blood has to maintain an acid level between 7.35 and 7.45 at all times. On a scale from 0 to 14, 7 is a neutral acid level. Anything below 7 is considered acidic and anything above 7 in considered alkaline. This makes our blood just slightly alkaline. Your lungs are the main organ which controls your pH levels in your blood. This is regulated by the intake of carbon dioxide. The less carbon dioxide we take in, the less acidic our blood will be and visa versa. If our blood dips above or below these acceptable levels, death or organ failure can occur. This is an extremely fine line between life and death. If your lungs can't handle the increase acidic condition, your kidneys take over and try to excrete the excess acid. This process becomes extremely difficult on your kidneys, which can cause kidney failure over a prolonged period of time. Overall, alkalinity is much healthier than being acidic. Most of our pH related health issues are attributed to an overly acidic condition call acidosis.

Primarily, acidosis is caused by an overabundance of acidic foods and beverages along with breathing too much carbon dioxide. Although our blood pH levels must remain between the acceptable levels, our cells tend to take the abuse associated with these elevated acidic conditions. As mentioned earlier, organ damage can occur along with other conditions such as gout and rheumatoid arthritis.

Elevated acid levels can cause your energy levels to decrease substantially. You may experience muscle pain and an overall feeling of discomfort. By changing your diet and air, this condition can be remedied over a period of time. The damage created by poor diet and air didn't occur overnight. Therefore, the repair may also take some time, up to six months in some instances. Some of this damage is permanent, especially with rheumatoid arthritis. Some of the pain will subside and the inflammation will decrease, but the joint damage will still exist. In the long term, a nutritionist is much more valuable for your overall health than any doctor.

To avoid contracting any of these acid based illnesses, your diet needs to consist of foods with high water content, such as fruit and vegetables. Soybeans, which should be omitted from our diets anyway, are very acidic. Most processed foods, meats, alcohol beverages, bread, and cheeses are highly acidic. Most oils, nuts, beans and dried fruits are neutrally balanced, which is fine for consumption. One of the most acidic food combinations to eat are cheeseburgers and French fries. Just think how many billions of these meals are eaten each year. If you happen to eat highly acidic foods, counterbalance your diet to include some very alkaline foods, as well. The Mexican diet is balanced in this very manner. The diet is overloaded with meat, rice, and beans. While meat is very acidic, the rice and beans are considered neutral. To counterbalance the acidic meat, lemon or lime is added to the meat to effectively turn the meat into an alkaline food. By nature, the salsas are very alkaline. The overall grade for this diet is slightly alkaline. The

Mexican people have lower cancers rates than most other cultures and the same holds true for the Japanese. The western diet is extremely overloaded with acidic foods, which correspond to higher rates of cancer, rheumatoid arthritis, gout, and organ failure. If small dietary changes were made to the western diet, such as having a salad or steamed vegetables with our steak, these illnesses could be prevented.

Some special preventive measures can change the alkalinity of our diet, such as using alkaline water, lemon/lime juice or apple cider vinegar. While overhyped, alkaline water can help our blood pH levels a little. What makes this water less effective is when we drink it, the water goes in an acid environment. This water basically neutralizes the effectiveness of our stomach acid. If we drink this water on an empty stomach, we can see minor health benefits. If we drink the water with food, our stomach acid will not be able to perform its duty very effectively. Lemon/lime juice and apple cider vinegar are much more effective at creating an alkaline environment. Since these ingredients are acidic by nature, by adding these liquids to our stomach acid, it creates an ideal acidic situation in our stomach. Since both lemon/lime juice and apple cider vinegar help break down our foods, similar to our stomach acid, they aid in our digestion process. In Chapter 15, all the health benefits associated with apple cider vinegar will be further explained.

Along with a sugar based diet and a lack of oxygen, cancer also thrives in an acid environment. If we create an alkaline situation, cancer can't survive similar to stopping its sugar supply and increasing our oxygen levels. This is the main reason an alkaline diet is so important. If our cells become high in alkalinity, cancer will not have a place to fester. Therefore, we will never contract this disease. Since we talked about lowering our blood pH levels, let talk a little about lower our cell pH levels as well.

In order to bring our cell pH levels to an alkaline state, we must continually keep our blood pH levels at a consistently low level. This can become extremely tricky, since having our pH levels too low in our blood can cause a fatal condition called alkalosis. When our blood pH levels become too low, our lungs will slow down our oxygen flow. This action causes the carbon dioxide levels to increase in our blood to counterbalance the increased alkalinity. This condition is just the opposite of acidosis, which we talked about earlier in the chapter. If we eat or drink too many alkaline foods and beverages, alkalosis can occur. The warning sign is the slowness of breath. If you experience this condition, it would be advisable to eat some acidic foods immediately after feeling such symptoms. This is a rare condition caused mainly by an individual who is trying to intentionally bring down their acid levels too quickly. As an example, a person drinking a glass of apple cider vinegar a couple times a day and eating a vegan diet will surely develop alkalosis. By being aware of the acid content in our foods, use your common sense and try to keep your pH levels on the low end of the pH scale. Eventual your cells will turn to an alkaline state. If you already have cancer or have had it in the past, make sure your pH levels remain lower than normal. A vegetarian diet is recommended for all cancer patients.

CHAPTER 10:
This Diet Doesn't Have Pills?

ARE PILLS REALLY NEEDED for a diet? The answer is no. My interpretation of a diet means food, liquids, air, and exercise. This chapter will educate you on the use of several vitamins, minerals, and herbs which can prevent certain illnesses and help with weight loss. Overall, eating foods with natural nutrients should be your primary focus. If your body is healthy by eating the right foods, breathing quality air, drinking the right liquids along with the proper exercise, why would you need diet pills? Quick-fix diet pills create an unhealthy environment and ultimately cause excessive weight gain. By putting the correct nutrients into our bodies and producing lean muscle mass, the weight you lose will never come back. Say goodbye to the old you and say hello to the new person you will become. When you achieve health from the inside out, others will see your transformation in a new light.

During this chapter, I will review many of the critical vitamins and minerals to explain their value and where to find them in our foods. If these items are too hard to locate through our food supply, you may feel enticed to purchase certain supplements. Otherwise, every nutrient can be found in our food, fluids, and air. Let's begin with vitamins.

Vitamin A: Carrots, sweet potatoes, kale and other dark leafy vegetables are all high in this powerful anti-oxidant.

Vitamin B1 (Thiamin): Fish, pork and most seeds are high in this cell and organ supporting nutrient.

Vitamin B2 (Riboflavin): Goat cheese, almonds, nuts, and beef are high in this energy metabolizing and cell supporting nutrient.

Vitamin B3 (Niacin): Fish, chicken, turkey and pork are high in the fat burning, cholesterol regulating and blood sugar regulating nutrient.

Vitamin B5: (Pantothenic Acid): Mushrooms, cheese, and oily fish are high in this fat maintaining and cell supporting nutrient.

Vitamin B6: Sunflower seeds, pistachio nuts, bananas, and fish are high in the red blood cell, nervous and immune system supporting nutrient.

Vitamin B9 (Folate): Beans, lentils, and spinach are high in this cell supporting nutrient.

Vitamin B12: Shellfish, beef liver, and mackerel are high in this very complex nutrient.

Vitamin B17 (Laetrile): Plum, peach and apricot pits are high is this powerful cancer-fighting nutrient.

Vitamin C (Absorbic Acid): Oranges, red peppers, kale, Brussels sprouts, and broccoli are high in this powerful anti-oxidant.

Vitamin D: The sun, cod liver oil and mushrooms are high in this calcium absorbing, bone developing, immune system supporting and inflammation fighting nutrient.

Vitamin E: Almonds, raw seeds, and dark leafy greens are high is this powerful anti-oxidant,

Vitamin K: Basil, green leafy vegetables, and scallion onions are high in this protein supporting and blood clotting nutrient.

Minerals are just as critical, if not more critical than vitamins at achieving a healthy well-being. These elements make up about 5% of our total body weight. If not for minerals, our bones, teeth, nerves, blood, skin, hair, muscle and energy production would be severely affected. Here is a list of all the critical minerals along with their food sources and function. We will start with the major minerals.

Sodium: Salt and processed foods are high in this water regulating, nerve transmitting and muscle contracting mineral. This mineral is one of the critical electrolytes needed during exercise. Most people eat an overabundance of this mineral.

Chloride: Salt and processed foods are high in this fluid balancing and stomach acid supporting mineral. This mineral comes from the same source as sodium and is also an electrolyte.

Potassium: Meats, cheese, fruit, vegetables, grains, and legumes are all high in this fluid regulating, nerve transmitting and muscle contracting electrolyte mineral.

Calcium: Milk products, green vegetables, and legumes are high in this bones and teeth maintaining, blood pressure regulating, muscle supporting, immune system supports, blood clotting and nerve transmitting electrolyte mineral.

Phosphorus: Meats, fish, eggs and milk are high in this teeth, bones, and cell supporting mineral, which also helps maintain our pH balance, as well.

Magnesium: Nuts, seeds, legumes and green leafy vegetable are high in this protein synthesizing, nerve and muscle supporting electrolyte mineral, which also supports the immune system and is critical for digestion.

Sulfur: Meats, eggs, milk products, nuts, and legumes are high in this protein supporting mineral.

Though we may need smaller amounts of these trace minerals, their significance is just as important to maintain a healthy being. Here is a list of trace minerals, along with their source and function.

Iron: Organ meats, eggs, green leafy vegetables, legumes and dried fruit are high in this critical red blood cell and oxygen supporting mineral which also aids in energy production.

Zinc: Meats, whole grain, and vegetables are high in this enzyme, protein and genetic supporting mineral which also help to heal wounds, aid in sperm production and helps with general sexual health along with is an immune system supporter.

Iodine: Seafood, seaweed, and iodized salt are high in this thyroid and cell supporting mineral.

Selenium: Meats, seafood, and grains are high in the power anti-oxidizing mineral with tremendous cancer preventing properties.
Copper: Legumes, seeds, nuts, whole grains and organ meat are high in this enzyme supporting and iron metabolizing mineral.
Manganese: Plant-based foods are high in the enzyme supporting mineral.
Fluoride: Drinking water and fish are high in this bones and tooth-damaging poison and man-made mineral.
Chromium: Beef liver, whole grains, nut, and cheese are high in the blood sugar regulating mineral.
Molybdenum: Legumes, grains, and green leafy vegetables are high in this enzyme supporting mineral.

Many herbs and spices have tremendous healing powers. Some of these items have been known throughout time as nature's medicine. Here is a list of some of the most popular herbs and spices with healing and supportive properties. If you have a condition, no doubt a herb can relieve the symptoms. Up until the invention of prescription drugs, herbs were the medicine of choice. Here are a few of the most popular herbal medicines and their function.

Bilberry: Used to increase the circulation to the eyes.
Black Cohosh: Used to treat menopausal symptom and relieve arthritis pain.
Cinnamon: Used for weight loss and for better sugar metabolizing.
Dandelion Root: Used to boost liver function and acts as an anti-oxidant and anti- inflammatory.
Echinacea: Used as an immune system booster.
Elderberry: Used as an antiviral remedy.
Garlic: Used as a powerful antimicrobial and blood pressure regulator, also used for yeast infections.
Ginger: Used as a probiotic, for nausea, and also cold and flu reliever.

Gingko Biloba: Used to increase brain and memory function.
Ginseng: Used to relieve mental and physical stress, immune
     booster, energy booster and to treat erectile dysfunction.
Kava: Used to relieve anxiety and as a muscle relaxer.
Milk Thistle: Used to support liver and kidney function.
St. John's Wort: Used to treat depression, sleep disorders
     and menopausal issues.
Turmeric: Used for almost everything imaginable. From
weight loss to chemo and radiation poisoning during cancer
treatments, Turmeric is probably the best herb for general
     health.

The medicinal uses for many foods are tremendous just as
other foods have destructive powers. Education and awareness
are the greatest tools regarding our health. Subconsciously,
these two tools can make a huge difference. Even if you read
this book as fiction, deep inside your eating habits will slightly
change. Let's talk a little about medicinal foods. Here is a list
of some of the best preventive and healing foods.

Apricots: Used to prevent kidney stones.
Banana: Is rich in Vitamin B6, which aids in serotonin levels
     for improved mental health.
Cabbage: Used as a hormone balancer and has the ability to
     heal stomach ulcers.
Carrots: Used as a cure for cancer and eye health.
Cranberry: Used for urinary tract illnesses and overall
     kidney health.
Grapes: Used for all facets of cardiovascular health.
Honey: Used to balance hormones and is a powerful
     anti-oxidant.
Pears: Used to fight high bad cholesterol.
Potato: Used to relieve tension headaches.

If you notice a certain nutrient is impossible to acquire through food, you may feel compelled to purchase a certain supplement. I am not opposed to such a purchase, especially in regards to the herbs. However, most vitamins and minerals should be obtained through food. I personally take many herbal supplements, such as bilberry, gingko biloba, and turmeric on a daily basis. All the natural nutrients obtained through food are much healthier and better absorbed than artificial supplements since most of these vitamins and minerals supplements are chemical based. Remember, we are trying to eliminate such chemicals. If you develop an ailment which requires an enormous amount of a certain nutrient, I encourage the use of such supplements until the ailment is relieved. For instance, vitamin C and zinc are two of the most useful healers known to humankind. These two nutrients can be more powerful than any antibiotic given by your doctor. Through food, it would be nearly impossible to acquire enough of these nutrients to cure a certain illness. However, with supplements, a high dosage can be achieved. The best part about The Infinity Diet is you'll rarely be sick since your liver and immune system will be running at peak performance on a daily basis. Your super white blood cells will destroy any viruses or infections before they can fester into something more serious.

CHAPTER 11:

So You Need To Learn How To Cook

COOKING CAN BE A WONDERFUL experience for some and a total burden for others. For this diet to fully work, you will need to learn some basic cooking skills. Since our food supply is so tainted, eating out every meal is definitely not your best option. For instance, if you happen to eat out for breakfast, do you know if your eggs were cooked in GMO soybean oil in a Teflon coated pan and laid by GMO fed chickens? Sometimes what appears to be healthy is just an illusion.

At home, we can control our ingredients and cooking processes. Each facet is critical to our well-being. In earlier chapters, we touched on the subject of using quality ingredients and talked a little about cookware. Let's expand on this subject of cookware, since using quality ingredients should be common sense more than an education.

The two healthiest forms of cookware appear to be ceramic and cast iron. Each form of this cookware can also have some risk. With ceramic cookware, some of the cheaper brands use a lead based glaze to protect the cooking surface. This glaze can leach into the food, causing neurological damage over a prolonged period of time. I would suggest doing some research to find the healthiest ceramic cookware possible. Many of the brands advertise their manufacturing processes as a marketing tool to further their sales. This information is invaluable when purchasing quality pots and pans.

Although a few risks are associated with cast iron cookware, overall this cookware has tremendous health benefits. The benefit of cast iron is the metal leaches a well-absorbed type of iron into our digestive system. If you happen to be anemic, cast iron should be your only form of cookware. I prefer using cast iron cookware due to the taste of the food. The taste associated with these pots and pans is extraordinary. This cookware appears to bring out the natural flavors more than any other cookware. Cast iron does require maintenance and special care. The pots and pans should never be washed, if possible. If washed, this cookware should be heated immediately to dissipate the moisture and coated with cooking oil soon afterward. This cookware also collects carbon. Carbon is a byproduct of everything we burn. Since carbon is a carcinogen (cancer causing agent), use extreme caution while cooking. Do not disturb the cooking surface. This will cause the baked-on carbon to flake off into your food.

Teflon, aluminum and stainless steel cookware should be avoided. As explained earlier, aluminum has been associated with such neurological disorders as Parkinson's disease, Alzheimer's disease, and dementia. Stainless steel contains a heavy metal named chromium, which can cause an array of serious illnesses. Chromium, in its metal form, is very toxic to the human body. Teflon is derived from the plastics industry. This substance is extremely toxic and has been linked to several different types of cancer.

Barbequing and smoking our foods is extremely toxic to the human body. The fumes contain carbon particles, which embed into to our foods. As explained earlier in this chapter, carbon is a cancer causing agent. I understand the flavor is tremendous, but so are the health risks.

Using a gas stove and oven is much more cost efficient, yet relatively unhealthy. The gas fumes contain toxins which leach into our foods. Though not nearly as harmful as barbecuing or smoking, we should try to keep as many toxins away from our bodies as possible. Health and longevity should continue being your driving force over taste and pleasure.

Microwave cooking should be avoided for several reasons. The oven itself uses a small dose of radiation to heat our food. Since radiation has been linked to thyroid issues and cancer, microwave ovens should be avoided. If you choose to use one of these ovens, always put your food in glass or non-lead glazed ceramic. By using plastic cookware, the petroleum-based chemicals in the plastic will leach into our foods. Plastic has been linked to cancer, sterility and a host of other illnesses. Tests have shown that microwave popcorn can cause male sterility and birth defects. The bag used to heat microwavable popcorn contains a chemical that produces this terrible effect.

Electricity appears to be the cleanest form of cooking. Since no fumes or radiation is used to heat the food, electricity is the only logical choice. I recently started using an induction stove. The burner is amazing because it heats the food extremely fast and efficiently. Crockpots are wonderful too since they are made from ceramic and use electricity for their heating element. The feature I love most about crockpots is their simplicity. Any busy person can cook healthy meals without any excuses. Simply wash some vegetables, season some meat and throw all the ingredients in the pot, put the setting on low and go to work. When you arrive after a long day, dinner is ready. It's that easy. It's a 10 minute prepped dinner with leftovers for lunch the next day.

To be a good cook, you have to use your imagination and understand the taste of the ingredients. When we were children, we mixed mud with rocks and sticks to make a mess. As adults, we mixed lettuce, cabbage, cucumbers, carrots, tomatoes and dressing to make a salad. We learned that combining different ingredients we could create something, good, bad or indifferent. So I like to think of cooking as a chemistry class for food. If we combine the wrong ingredients, we might have a dud. However, if we mix the right ingredients, we could make magic. One general rule is if you decide to use a bitter or sour, always include a sweet. The contrasting flavors each compliment the other to make your taste buds come alive. A good example is combining a little lime juice with apple juice. Usually sour or bitter is overpowering, so don't add too much lime juice. Try this at home, if you get a chance.

Marinara sauce is a great example of combining ingredients to make magic. The base starts with tomatoes. Buy a bunch of tomatoes and lightly boil them until just slightly tender. Drain the water and peel the tomatoes. After the tomatoes are peeled, smash them into chunks. You just made stewed tomatoes. Now your creativity can begin since you finished the base. To give your sauce flavor, I like to add finely chopped garlic and onion.

These ingredients will give the sauce a tangy bite. The garlic will give it a big kick, while the onion gives the sauce a more subtle taste. To increase the flavor, I like to add oregano. Oregano gives the sauce that classic Italian flavor. If you like sweet, add some basil. Basil mixed with oregano is a subtle blend of sour and sweet to give your sauce a wonderful flavor. Sometimes if I'm in the mood, I will add one deseeded, finely chopped jalapeno pepper to the sauce for a hint of spice. Other times, I will cut up a red or yellow bell pepper and add a little extra basil to make the sauce even sweeter. Another time, I may add a green bell pepper and extra oregano to give the sauce a stronger kick. Another ingredient you can add is celery to make the sauce slightly salty. Some people like to add olive oil to bring down the taste. Others like to add a little red wine to add a mild punch or ground pepper for added spiciness. Taste each component by itself and sample the sauce in between ingredients. This experiment is fun and will give you a better understanding of how to create food.

While you were making the sauce, take a spaghetti squash and cut it in half. Rub a combination of olive oil and garlic powder on the inside of each half of the squash. Put the squash back together and wrap the entire squash in foil. Preheat the oven to 350 degrees. Cook the squash for 35-40 minutes, until soft. Now you have created an extremely nutritious meal at around 100 calories per serving. Remember, your body only cares about nutrients, not calories.

Soups are also fun and nutritious to make. A pot of soup can last the family for days and is extremely inexpensive to make. First, determine what kind of base you're craving. There are a couple different bases to choose from, tomato or natural with salt. I like to determine which protein to use at the same time as determining my base. I usually pick between beans, chicken or beef. Pork soup is a little strange for my taste buds, so I avoid using pork. If you choose beans as your protein, soak the beans overnight to soften them first. This will make the beans much more palatable.

To start the soup, I begin with the protein. If you plan to use meat in your soup, make sure to buy meat with bones. If you decide on chicken or turkey, use the skin. The skin will add more flavor to your soup. The bone marrow is fantastic for your health and adds a tremendous amount of flavor. In the beginning, start with half a pot of water and the protein. I like to add a quartered onion, a few bay leaves and a clove or two of crushed garlic into the broth for seasoning. Bring to a boil, and then reduce the heat to simmer for about a half an hour. Next is to add the other seasonings, such as bullion for the salty taste or crushed tomatoes, oregano and basil for a tomato base. If I use a tomato base, I usually don't add salt. I only use the natural herbs and spices. Next, I add the hard vegetables, such as carrots, corn, and chayote squash. Bring back to a boil, and again reduce the heat to a simmer, until the vegetables are slightly soft. After the hard vegetables soften a little, I like to add the rest of the vegetables, such as celery, potatoes, various squashes, cabbage, green beans or jalapeno peppers. Bring back to a boil, and then reduce again to a simmer. If you decide to use a tomato base, you can squeeze a lemon into the broth right before the potatoes become soft for an added zing. The potatoes are the indicator if the soup is ready. If the potatoes become soft through to the center, your soup is done. At around 150 calories per bowl, this is a wonderfully nutritious meal for the whole family to enjoy.

When it comes to healthy cooking, owning a crock pot or cast iron Dutch oven is the best investments one can make. Like explained early, a crock pot is the easiest, yet healthiest, way to cook. The same can be said about a Dutch oven, except you have to be present in order to cook with this cookware. Again, select a cut of bone-in meat and season with whatever your taste buds desire. Some of my favorite seasonings are turmeric, garlic and balsamic vinegar with lemon juice, depending on my mood. With chicken, I normally pick turmeric. I will sprinkle the chicken with spices and place the meat in the crockpot on the low setting. With a Dutch oven, I place the seasoned meat at the bottom of the oven, replace the cover and set the stove on a medium setting. As the meat starts to heat, the natural juices will be released. The vegetables will be steamed in these same juices. With pork and beef, I prefer using onion and garlic powder as my seasonings. Pepper can also make a wonderful seasoning and the taste is fantastic. When I prepare beef, I sometimes use balsamic vinegar and lemon as a tenderizer. The taste and texture of the meat will melt in your mouth. With the crock pot, put the vegetables in with the meat and forget about it for several hours until the meat in thoroughly cooked and tender. With the Dutch oven, wait until the meat is almost done and add the vegetables right on top of the meat, just like the crock pot. I like to use the same vegetables as in my soup recipe, except for adding sweet potatoes. You can add whatever vegetables you like since this is your meal. Trying new things makes cooking fun. Remember; treat cooking like a science experiment for the palette. Each of these meals will be around 250 calories per serving

I consider green salads as a form of cooking. Any cold vegetable can be used for salad, such as avocados, tomatoes, cucumbers, lettuce, cabbage, onions, broccoli, cauliflower, bell peppers, sweet peppers, carrots, kale, cactus, and radishes. Several fruits can also be added, such as apples and berries to make new creations. Fruit salads are also wonderful, but higher in calories due to the added sugar content. Nuts and seeds are a wonderful, crunchy addition to any creation. Some common salad nuts and seeds are pine nuts, sunflower seeds, almond slivers, walnuts, and cashews.

When it comes to salad dressings, try to avoid the ready-made products. If you happen to read the labels, most of these high-calorie dressings contain high fructose corn syrup, soybean oil and an array of chemicals. If you create your own dressing, you're assured the ingredients are healthy. The easiest dressing to make is vinegar and oil. There are many varieties of vinegar and oils in which to choose from. My personal favorite is balsamic vinegar and olive oil, with crushed garlic, onion powder, and oregano. This simple dressing can also be used as a marinade for some of your meat dishes. Another dressing I like to make is apple cider vinegar, lemon juice, basil and onion powder. This zero calorie dressing tastes great and has tremendous health benefits. As you will learn in chapter 15, apple cider vinegar is one of the greatest substances we can consume.

Try to avoid the mayonnaise based dressings. These dressings are extremely high in calories and bad fats. If you happen to dislike vinegar dressings, use the other dressings sparingly. I like to use a small amount of the dressing and shake the salad so it is evenly dispersed throughout the contents.

Another wonderful dish is zucchini, crushed tomatoes, and onions with garlic and oregano. This extremely low-calorie dish can be prepared in 20 minutes. Simply cut the ingredients, except the zucchini and add to a pan on medium heat, stirring continuously until the tomatoes are turned into chunks. Add the zucchini last and reduce the heat to low and cover. The tomato juice will soften the zucchini and create a wonderful dish.

All type of steamed vegetables can easily be made and are tremendous for your health. From artichokes to carrots, all steamed vegetables should be consumed on The Infinity Diet. Just add a couple of tablespoons of good oil to your water, and steam away. These easily made foods are very low in calories and extremely high in nutrients. Steaming preserves most of the nutrients within the vegetables, while boiling releases many of the nutrients into the water. By adding a little oil to your water prior to steaming, your vegetables won't require butter or any other condiment to enhance the flavor. I usually top my vegetables with little pepper and enjoy. I also try not to add any salt to my food since most foods are already laden by this mineral.

For breakfast, I like to make eggs and vegetables for a healthy meal. This simple and fast breakfast is a great way to start your day. Eggs are a wonderful source of protein and the

Vegetables will kickstart your day with the needed complex carbs. I like to use coconut oil as my non-sticking agent due to its extreme health benefits. Our body also needs healthy fat in the morning for energy. I usually add a half of avocado on top of my creation for even more fat and nutrients. By making breakfast your highest calorie meal of the day, your body will be assured of all the proper nutrients and calories needed to successfully start your metabolism. Some of the vegetables I like to add to my eggs are cactus, tomatoes, onions, broccoli, spinach, zucchini and peppers of all varieties. A two egg breakfast with a various combination of ingredients will contain about 600 calories. Your lunch, snacks, and dinner should contain about another 1,000 calories from the meal ideas I described earlier in this chapter. Remember, your body needs nutrients, not calories. The calories are on your butt, thighs, and stomach.

What is the difference between designing a toaster and creating a wonderful dish? Each has a bunch of components which do little until they are combined to make something special. Try to experience new tastes from a bunch of ingredients and have fun with them. If one of your creations tastes bad, I hope you have a dog. Usually, your dog will eat anything. If not, try the kids. The look on their faces should make your life a little more enjoyable.

I hope this chapter was fun for you. Since I'm a foodie at heart, I really enjoyed writing about the different ways to prepare food. Being a former engineer, cooking is a healthy outlet for me. I can still create and enjoy the fruits of my labor.

CHAPTER 12:
You Mean I Can Cheat !!!

WITH HUMAN NATURE, EVERYONE has the tendency to stray off their chosen path from time to time. This is a quality that many of us have a hard time accepting. With this diet, cheating is encouraged. Small changes in our lives keep us from boredom. I feel if you veer off once in a while, the daunting task of eating correctly will become less cumbersome. The funniest part is your body wants you to stray occasionally too. A pizza here and a burger and fries there won't kill you. It may give you indigestion, but it won't kill you. My guilty pleasure is ice cream. Since I rarely eat this food, I will binge eat a whole half gallon for dinner. Oh, it tastes so good. Should I feel bad because I ate this? Absolutely not. The last time I checked I was human too. I tell this story to some of my clients and they freak out. "How can you do that to your body being a nutritionist?" is the common question. My answer is without pleasure, what good is living? As much as I preach about finding different pleasure outlets other than food, I believe on occasions it is perfectly acceptable to use your tongue as a pleasure center. The problem is distinguishing between cheating and creating a habit. If you cheat on your diet, don't begin eating badly again on a consistent basis. When cheating becomes a habit, you have fallen off track. You may have to read this book again or use your willpower to get yourself back on your path. I fall off occasionally too. I'm human. The main thing is to get back on track and not veer too far away. The overall goal is to live a long and healthy life. Eating pizza and burgers will not achieve this goal.

In the previous paragraph, I said cheating is good for the body. This is true. When we eat something out of our normal realm of food, our body considers it as poison. After several months of eating The Infinity Diet, your body will rid itself of most of the byproducts leftover from your previous diet. I suggest to my clients to eat something laden with bad fat after about six months of eating correctly to create this poisoning effect. A pizza or a couple orders of French fries usually does the trick. When we eat this foreign substance, our body will reject this same material leftover within our system. It is typical to lose 3-5 pounds overnight on one binge eating spree. It is called shock. If you shock your body hard enough, all the leftover toxins from the same ingredients in your pizza or fries will be rejected too. For instance, you could have a bunch of cheese fat accumulated in your butt. When you eat the pizza, your body will try to locate this same type of poison throughout your body and flushes it out of your system. Now your butt just became smaller. It's advisable to have a terrible cheat meal once a month to keep your body off guard. As soon as your binge meal is over, go back to The Infinity Diet. When you resume your diet, your body will become more accepting of the nutrient-rich foods once again. I hope this makes sense to you. The human body sometimes defies all logic.

Here is a success story about my friend Al. Al is a personal trainer and sports nutritionist. He chose to take a high paying job as a loan officer to make more income than his training and nutrition business was creating. After a couple of years, his sit down job gave him diabetes and he had gained 80 pounds. Understanding health is more valuable than wealth, Al and his wife decided he should get back into the fitness business, but who would listen to a fat guy about nutrition and fitness? Anyhow, being knowledgeable and understanding what he needed to do to lose the weight, Al embarked on the path to health once again. Al started to exercise and watch what he was eating. In no time, Al had lost 60 lbs over a 4 month period and looked like a fitness guy once again. However, Al still wanted to lose that last 20 lbs, but his body became accustomed to the clean diet and he just couldn't lose the weight. Al had a hard time understanding how the body could stay the same weight with a calorie deficit. So he came to me for advice. I explained his body needed a shock to get back on track. So I pulled out my wallet and found a $10 bill. I told Al to buy a pizza and eat the whole thing. He became upset at me and said I was crazy. I told him to take my money, get a pizza and tell me how much weight he lost in the morning. Al said, "Damn it, I'm going to take your money and eat that f*cking pizza". The next morning he called me in shock. He explained that he ate all but one slice because he was full and he had lost 3 lbs overnight. Over the next month, he lost the 20 lbs he wanted to lose and got rid of his diabetes. Now every couple of weeks, he binge eats something out of the ordinary to shock his body back into shape. Al looks and feels great today and his business is thriving. I think his decision to take health over wealth probably saved his life. He now uses this principal with many of his clients who have become stagnant on their own diet. This just goes to prove that sometimes what we feel is right, is actually wrong, like cardio is in the exercise chapter.

Some people feel by breaking their diet for a day, it will cause them to gain a bunch of weight instantly. This is true to some extent. An Italian restaurant in my hometown has a 3 1/2 pound prime rib dinner on the first of every month. If you decide to eat that whole dinner, you will gain 3 1/2 pounds for a few days until your digestive system can process it. You might also gain a half a pound of fat because the meat will slow down your metabolism. In reality, it takes 3,500 calories over your metabolic rate to gain one pound of fat. Otherwise, if a woman who utilizes 2,000 calories a day decided to eat 3,000 calories instead, she will gain about 1/4 of a pound for that day. If she continues to eat these extra calories for a whole year, she will gain about 90 lbs. On the other hand, if this same woman reduces her calorie intake to 1,500 calories per day eating highly nutritious foods, she will lose about 1/8 of a pound a day or about 45 lbs for the year. What if she happened increases her metabolism through proper exercise to 2,500 calories and continues to eat 1,500 calories, she will lose 1/4 of a pound per day or 90 lbs for the year. Everybody thinks weight loss is so difficult when actually, it is simple arithmetic and eating the correct foods.

Do you think if you binge eat every once in a while you will become fatter? The answer is no for two reasons.

The first reason is your body will reject the food and other related substances as poison after the binge. The second reason is, so what if you eat an extra 1,000 calories today if you remain on your path to health. This is so true. Being consistent with your diet is the main factor. A blip here or there isn't going to change anything. When you eat a nutritious, low-calorie diet, these brief dietary changes have no effect whatsoever on weight gain.

Your only concern is to avoid chemical laden foods during your cheat days. Try to prepare your own cheat meals since you have no idea what quality of food you will be purchasing. A home-made pizza is a wonderful cheat meal and is also fun to make. In the previous chapter, we created our own pizza sauce, so we can skip this ingredient. The crust can be purchased at your local grocery store which will be bad due to the issues with today's wheat. The cheese, by far, is the worst ingredient in the pizza. Try to buy organic mozzarella cheese and toppings. This will be a fun project and try to get your whole family involved. To start, a large cheese pizza is around 2,000 calories. Some of the toppings like sausage and pepperoni are full of calories and not very good for you.

Fried mozzarella sticks are also horribly unhealthy. You can make them with cheese sticks, bread crumbs and fried in coconut or safflower oil. These sticks are also a great poison induced meal. I suggest having this meal on the weekend since you shouldn't have school or work the next day. At times, you may not feel well afterward. If you are lactose intolerant, donuts or a pie are full of bad fats and can cause the same poisoning effect. Tamales are a great poison too, especially cheese tamales. Since the masa is made with lard, the body will tend to reject any bad animal fats you have accumulated over the years.

If you chose The Infinity Diet for maintenance purposes and you decide to stay focused on health, cheating is not required, it's an option. By remaining on track, your body will achieve a certain level of health and remain there until you expire. The cheating portion of this diet is for individuals who want to lose weight by shocking their systems. As effective as this may be, maintains a healthy, uninterrupted diet is equally beneficial. If you stay health conscientious with every meal, a slip here and there won't make any difference. Studies have shown if we maintain a healthy diet, all the damage caused by our previous unhealthy diet can be reversed. These words should be very encouraging.

Here's a little story about human resilience and how the body responses to falling off the wagon for a long period of time. I, myself fell off my wagon for 10 months by suffering a severe life altering event. I didn't care about anything, except for repairing my dilemma. I shoveled garbage into my mouth from every drive thru imaginable on a daily basis. I also didn't cook one single meal during this whole traumatic period. I had gained back 40 lbs and felt awful. My diabetes came back with a vengeance and my energy levels dropped like a rock. I didn't exercise and my body changed drastically. One day while visiting a local gym, one of the guys working out poked me in the stomach and said, "What kind of nutritionist are you? You're fat". I had to do one of the hardest things known to humankind, I had to stand and look at myself in the mirror. It's easy being critical of others, but looking at yourself is difficult. He was absolutely right. I had reverted to an unhealthy lifestyle and my mind and body were suffering for it. I didn't even realize how bad I had gotten because repairing my life became more important than maintaining my health. I said to myself, "What good is living if your health is suffering?" With the desire to stop my path to self-destruction, I decided to make my health my second largest priority once again. Parenting will always be my first priority. So I jumped off my wagon of despair and started cooking and exercising once again. Then something amazing occurred. My personal problems began to disappear along with my stomach. By eating the right nutrients and allowing my body to produce the right endorphins, my thought process improved. I became a finely tuned machine once again, ready to handle whatever adversity may come my way. Did some of my personal problems still exist? Yes, however, I was able to think more clearly and come up with better solutions. In two months, I had lost 25 of the 40 lbs I had gained and my energy levels went back to the way they were previously. My diabetes reverted back to acceptable levels and I started to regain some of my stress-induced muscle loss. A few months later, I was back in the local gym when the same guy showed up. He couldn't poke me in the stomach this time and I wasn't there to visit, I was there to exercise.

I hope this personal story will give you some insight on how incredibly human we actually are. Almost every person has some kind of self-destructive tendencies or addictions they have to overcome. If you feel that your cheat meals may become addicting, don't cheat. Just like a smoker or an alcoholic, that one cigarette or drink can put you back on your self-destructive path once again. I should know. I quit smoking twice because I had one cigarette, which started up my addiction once more. Now I refuse if I'm offered.

If you have the willpower to resume your diet where you left off, you shouldn't have a problem. Have your cheat meals only when you become stagnant or have hit a plateau in your weight. One of the local gym owners had a client who went to a weight loss camp for three months. After about 6 months on his diet, he became stagnant and his weight remained the same. This owner called me and asked if I would meet with his client. I asked the client what was his guilty pleasure. He told me pastrami sandwiches with Swiss cheese and he hadn't had one of over 6 months. I explained to him about how cheating can get his body back on track. This client became very angry and started to cry. He told me if he ever had another pastrami sandwich, he would be doomed to fail once more. I realized he couldn't handle the cheat meal because he had food addiction issues. Anyway, who knows your body and mind better than you? If you can handle a cheat meal, cheat. If you can't, don't do it.

CHAPTER 13:

The Outside Factors

IF YOU HAVE SUCCESSFULLY made it this far reading this book, your tool box should be full. Maybe your brain has asked you to begin your new lifestyle. For those procrastinators in the world, you're only cheating yourself to live a long and healthy life. What irks me are the people who won't make small changes to receive huge rewards. To some, taste is more important than extending their lives for many extra years. I have even seen some individuals in tremendous pain choose taste over suffering. Personally, life is much more important to me than taste. Except for humans, All other animals on this planet eat to survive. Can you change your thought process? By eating a proper diet, your quality of life can improve dramatically. Isn't happiness and health more important than pain and unhappiness?

According to researchers, the human body is designed to live about 100 years. The oldest verified person lived to be about 122 and a half and the oldest unverified person was said to have lived to be 157. Many in the scientific community now believe humans could live to be 150 if we take very good care of ourselves and live in a clean environment. Unfortunately, the average life expectancy is decreasing due to several man-made factors. What should we expect in our future? With two catastrophic events about to severely decrease the world's life expectancy, I'm not sure what to expect in the very near future. I feel the best a person can do is to take precautionary measures to ensure their own life isn't severely affected. This may be an impossible task, but well worth a try since it is our own life we are trying to save. Time will only tell how large of a death toll these events will have on the world's population.

Based on historical records, a nuclear power plant was destroyed at Chernobyl in the Ukraine in 1986. This catastrophe took almost a million lives from 1986 to 2004. Statistics weren't kept after 2005 because it was too difficult to pinpoint the cause of death by radiation compared to natural occurring mortality. Many researchers have estimated 3 million lives will be lost from this one catastrophic event. Each and every one of us has a small portion of radiation in our bodies from this disaster since radiation is accumulated in our organs over time and little is released through our urine and feces, under normal circumstances.

In 2011, an earthquake and tsunami destroyed a nuclear power plant in Fukushima, Japan. Although this meltdown released less radiation than Chernobyl, the majority of the contamination was released into our water supply, while at Chernobyl, the radiation was emitted into the air. Since all living creatures depending on water as our main source for life, this event has a far more reaching effect on our immediate well-being. Since all the water is shared throughout the world, this one cataclysmic event will alter all life forms on this planet for at least 150 years. The worst part is the radiation leak is still continuing today in 2017. The operators of this power plant haven't been able to contain the radiation and it is still leaking into the Pacific Ocean and into our ground water. While some of this radioactive material will dissipate and will be re-absorbed back into the Earth, Cesium-137 will not. This material actually disperses very well into the water.

If a dime sized amount of Cesium-137 was released in New York City, the city would become inhabitable for a minimum of 30 years and become radiation free in 150 years. Unfortunately, all estimates indicate Fukushima has released the equivalent of 4,000 dimes of Cesium-137 into our water supply and counting since this contamination is still continuing today. Because most of this material was released into the Pacific Ocean, our sea creatures have taken the biggest hit from this catastrophe. On the West Coast of the United States, a variety of mutated fish and other wildlife have washed up on the shore. Several varieties of fish caught in Canada and the Washington state area have cancer tumors protruding from their bodies. For instance, the bluefin tuna used for many of our canned tunas, have reported extremely high amounts of radiation. As the ocean currents travel around the world, the contamination will continue to infiltrate to every far reaching place on this planet. Water comes in so many different forms. From the ice sheets of Antarctica to the clouds in the sky, water is the main lifeblood of this planet. The waters of the Pacific Ocean will evaporate and will transform into clouds. The accumulated water in the clouds will create rain and snow. The rain and melted snow will be retained into reservoirs and used by farmers and as drinking water. The farmers will raise their crops to be consumed by people and animals. The cows and pigs will also drink the same water we consume and this cycle will continue. From the ice cubes in our sodas to the glaciers in Greenland, all the water on Earth run on a continuous cycle of life. Unfortunately, this precious gift of life will now include a destructive factor, which will affect all of the Earth's inhabitants. Due to these two catastrophes, every living creature will take a portion of this radiation to their grave. It is part of the cleansing process of this planet. Eventually, all the contamination will be dispersed through all life forms and our future generations should continue to live relatively radiation-free. Ok, that was wishful thinking. With 430 other nuclear power plants currently still operating worldwide, when will the next catastrophe happen? Humankind hasn't learned from their mistakes, especially when money is involved.

We have had the knowledge and understanding since the dawn of civilization on what form of energy should power the world. It's that bright yellow thing in the sky that keeps this planet from freezing. Isn't the sun a much healthier way to boil water and charge our batteries? I believe after the 3 Mile Island incident in 1979, nuclear power plants should have been scrapped because of the potential life altering consequences that could arise. Now it has happened twice with substantially increased environmental damage at each event. At some point, the self-destructive nature of human beings needs to be corralled for the betterment of all living creatures. Like I explained in my preface, what good is money when everyone else is dead?

A surrounding 23-mile radius around Chernobyl has been deemed uninhabitable for the past 31 years. The area within 5 miles of the power plant has been designated to be uninhabitable for the rest of eternity. When the radiation levels decrease around the perimeter sometime in the future, residents will be allowed to resume life in this area. Much of the Ukraine and Belarus still have high levels of radiation leftover from this meltdown in 1986. These countries experience lower birth rates, increased stillborn births and birth defects, compared to the world average. The cancer rates remain very high with the most prevalent being thyroid and organ cancer. So what is Japan's solution to their radiation problem? The answer is practically nothing.

When the Fukushima catastrophe first occurred, the radioactive cloud was blown eastward over the Pacific Ocean. However, the winds shifted in the following days directing the cloud westward over Tokyo. Radioactive fallout was dumped right on top the largest city in the world. All of Tokyo should have been evacuated and decontaminated. This city of 38 million people is only 150 miles away from the initial radioactive explosion. Since this disaster, the citizens of Tokyo have started to feel the effects related to radiation poisoning, largely due to the contaminated food supply. By fishing in the radioactive waters and the produce being grown with a tainted water supply, many farmers and fisherman are fearful they are selling contaminated food to their countrymen. In reality, they are. The farmers are watering their crops with radioactive water and the fishermen are fishing in waters not suitable for life. Many sailors are reporting an area 1,000 mile eastward from the mainland as a dead zone in the ocean. The fish being caught outside this area have visible cancer tumors protruding from their mouths and gill area. Since radiation poisoning is an accumulated disease, it may take upwards of 30 years to see the real tragedy of this cataclysmic event, as it did for the victims of Hiroshima and Nagasaki during World War 2.

Since Japan has set up an inhabitable zone of only 13 miles around the initial site, this leads me to believe the government is not being truthful with their citizens. The official word from the government is to just smile and be happy. What kind of public service message is this? I can understand not intentionally trying to alarm the public, but smile and be happy? I feel it's the government's responsibility to inform their citizens of such health risks. This is their citizen's lives that hang in the balance. This type of response is common from many of the governments of the world when they face adversity. They add whipped cream, chocolate syrup and top their answers with a cherry trying to divert the real truth. I think people have the right to know what is really happening. Someday, one of these cover-ups will cause a civil war. If we use our common sense and look through the propaganda being fed to us through our media, maybe we can save ourselves. Again, the ignorant and gullible are the media targets as explained earlier in this book.

What can we do to protect ourselves from these present and future tragic events? Since we have no individual control over these catastrophes from occurring, I feel our best chance is to constantly rid our bodies of this radiation. Remember, it has to accumulate in order to harm us. The sun alone emits a tremendous amount of radiation to our planet, so our world is already radioactive. By these catastrophes adding more contamination to our bodies than should be allowed, detoxification seems like the only logical answer.

One of the ways we can stay one step ahead of this damage is to begin drinking distilled water. Since distilled water is void of any minerals, this water tends to collect radiation, metals, and minerals for elimination. While absorbing these other compounds, the kidneys flush out many of these substances through our urine, thus ridding our body of radiation.

There are also drawbacks to drinking distilled water. The first reason for concern is distilled water is very acidic. As explained in an earlier chapter, our bodies should remain slightly alkaline for proper health. The second drawback is distilled water eliminates all metals and minerals. Many of these elements are necessary for proper health, such as calcium, magnesium, iron, iodine and a host of other essential minerals. By drinking distilled water on a consistent basis, the minerals in our bones will become depleted causing an array of other illnesses such as osteoporosis, hypothyroidism, and osteoarthritis. By adopting a routine of drinking a gallon of distilled water once a week, you will receive the benefit of eliminating the radioactive material from your body without severely depleting your mineral supply. With The Infinity Diet, your body will have an abundance of nutrients to combat any mineral depletion you may experience while drinking the distilled water.

Another way to prevent radiation poisoning is to take an iodine supplement. The thyroid gland is our radiation regulator and iodine is the nutrient needed to support its function. One of the common cancers associated with radiation poisoning is thyroid cancer. If the thyroid is unable to properly regulate the radiation levels or if there is an overabundance of radiation, our thyroid may not be able to handle the load and cancer can occur. By supporting our thyroid function through the supplementation of iodine, our chances of contracting this deadly illness will greatly diminish.

Another compound typically used to collect radiation is Zeolite. Zeolite was originally derived from settled volcanic ash in the mid-1700's. Although Zeolite is most commonly used for chelating (see below), recent studies have shown Zeolite has only one purpose, to collect Cesium. It actually produces poor results collecting other heavy metals and radioactive toxins. Since we are only concerned with Cesium poisoning, Zeolite remains one of the better options for this purpose.

Another very effective way to eliminate radiation from our body is through chelation. Chelation (pronounced KEY'LATION) is the elimination of heavy metals through supplementation. Similar to the use of distilled water, chelation targets the metals and minerals for elimination by attaching these materials to certain chelating compounds. These compounds are then eliminated through our feces and urine. It is strongly recommended to take an essential mineral supplement while using this method. Not only will chelation rid your body of radiation, many other harmful heavy metals will also be eliminated at the same time, such as mercury, chromium, and lead. This wonderful tool is recommended a year prior to pregnancy to ensure the child born will not have the effects of autism. This process appears to help rid many of the symptoms of fibromyalgia, as well.

There are several ways to chelate your body. The most popular methods require such items as EDTA, cilantro, chlorella, spirulina and vitamin C. EDTA is a weak synthetic amino acid used by the food industry as a preservative. However, the health benefits of taking this substance as a supplement are tremendous. Not only does it bind and eliminate heavy metals and radiation from our bodies, it also cleans out our circulatory system of unwanted calcium and plaque. It worked in the similar fashion as L-Arginine, except it is less harsh on the system. Think of EDTA as Liquid Plumber for your circulatory system. The only side effect associated with EDTA is it also binds and eliminates all the good metals and minerals such as calcium, iron, magnesium, zinc and manganese. It is strongly recommended to take mineral supplements during the use of this powerful chelation tool.

When it comes to natural chelation, nothing works better than cilantro, chlorella, and spirulina. Cilantro is a herb used as a topping on most Mexican foods and salsas. This herb comes from the coriander family and is considered a super food. The phytonutrients and minerals in the magical herb are unparalleled. Not only is this wonderful herb extremely nutritious, it also works as a chelating tool to eliminate heavy metals and radiation from our bodies. If you like the taste of this pungent herb, by all means, eat as much as possible. There are no side effects related to the consumption of this tremendous gift of health.

Chlorella is a green algae originating from the coral reefs of Japan, which is extremely high in protein and has an array of other nutrients. This superfood is extremely unique. It can regenerate human cells through our DNA and RNA, which dictate our genetic patterns. Research has shown that combining cilantro with chlorella, the elimination of heavy metals and radiation poisoning can be eliminated by 80%. This remarkable amount of detoxification can be achieved by consuming these two simple items. Just by supplementing with chlorella and cilantro will allow you a tremendous health advantage over the rest of the population.

Spirulina is a very close cousin of chlorella. This blue/green bacteria consists of 70% protein and hosts an array of valuable nutrients. Spirulina is very unique. This compound is only missing one component to replicate our red blood cells. So let's name this a super blood food. These amazing bacteria can also eliminate the heavy metals and radiation that gather throughout our lifetime. If we combine this superfood with chlorella and/or cilantro, this mixture can repair any damage within our bodies. AARP has labeled spirulina as the #1 life-prolonging food in the world and the United Nations has labeled spirulina as the cure for malnutrition.

Vitamin C is not only a powerful antioxidant, it can also bind and remove heavy metals and radiation found in our bodies. A very high dosage is required to reap these benefits, which can be taxing on the kidneys. If you have kidney issues, I suggest using one of the methods shown earlier in this chapter. The dosage required for chelation purposes is 5 to 10 grams a day. Normally only 30% of the vitamin C is absorbed through our intestines. I suggest taking this nutrient with a teaspoon of baking soda. By combining the ascorbic acid from the vitamin C with sodium bicarbonate in the baking soda, this transforms this composition into sodium absorbate. This nutrient is more easily absorbed into our bodies. Tests have shown sodium absorbate has an absorption rate of around 70%. Some precautions should be followed regarding the use of baking soda. Since baking soda is part of the sodium family, try to limit other salty foods during your chelation period. An overdose of salt can cause issues with water retention and blood pressure, just to name a few. Baking soda is also very alkaline. Do not combine any of the other alkalinity tools mentioned in chapter 9, such as apple cider vinegar with sodium bicarbonate. This combination could decrease your blood acid levels too low and cause alkalosis, also explained in chapter 9. Anyway, remember what happens when we combine vinegar and baking soda, what do we get? That's right, an explosion. Just remember your volcano science project in elementary school. This is not good for your physical well-being.

In regards to our health, baking soda is a pretty amazing product. This amazing substance is the best anti-fungal and anti- bacterial medicine known to humankind. For less than a dollar, baking soda can kill athlete's foot and most other microbe related illness including cancer, yes cancer!!!! Do you think your doctor would prescribe baking soda as a cancer treatment? I doubt it. One doctor did and he spent many years in jail. You can read about his story is in chapter 15. At the price of baking soda, your doctor's vacation home in Hawaii would be a grass hut.

I hope you heed this warning about the imminent environmental issues we face in today's world. With the cancer rates about to skyrocket, do you want to be one of those statistics?

Prevention is the key to living a long and healthy life. How long do you propose to live if you don't take this warning seriously? Although, we may have compassion for the sick and elderly, do we want this for ourselves? I would rather go to someone else's funeral than attend mine own. A good maintenance and preventive plan should keep us out of the mortuary for a very long time.

CHAPTER 14:
Is Your Peach Really A Peach?

AS A KID, I REMEMBER food tasting so good. We lived in a small town surrounded by orchards and fields. My grandmother and I also planted our own garden in the backyard and our whole family ate the fruits of our labor. Our friends and neighbors used to exchange their produce for ours. This gave both our families a wide variety of wonderful fruits and vegetables. The local farmers took very good care of their crops and use to share their produce with us, as well. I never saw a crop duster spraying pesticides on their fields, as a kid.

My grandparents owned a meat market, so the exchange of food would take place rather frequently. When we wanted eggs, we would drive to this lady's ranch that raised chickens. Her chickens were raised in huge rooms, where the poultry could roam free. She would walk around petting one of her chickens. I thought she raised the happiest chickens in the world.

When we wanted milk, we would go to a dairy farm. The dairy sold us milk in glass bottles. I was able to experience the whole process from milking the cow to pasteurization. The farmer actually allowed me to milk one of the cows on several occasions.

We also ate meat from wild animals. Usually, a family friend would go hunting and bring us a duck or a few quail. My grandmother would cook something tasty out of these animals. One of my favorites was deer meat. Venison is very sweet and it tastes wonderful made into jerky. Occasionally, someone would kill a wild boar. Since these animals are in the pig family, their meat tasted like the best pork you could ever imagine. The bacon was so savory and not nearly as fatty. Eating eggs from the lady's farm and wild boar bacon for breakfast made life good and very tasty.

I moved to the big city of Los Angeles when I was 13 years old, with my mother and sister. The first big change I noticed was breathing bad air and eating store bought food. Although the food tasted alright, it didn't have that just picked flavor I appreciated from my small town. My mother was a good cook, so she made the food taste better than it actually was. Boy did I miss the roadside produce stands and garden fresh vegetables.

Today with the mass population and our capitalistic society, do we really know what were eating? Like the title of the chapter says, is your peach really a peach? It may look like a peach, but it sure doesn't taste or acts like one. What kind of so-called foods are we being forced to eat? I remember when I ate a peach, I needed a napkin because it was so juicy and the flavor would jump onto my taste buds. I recently bought some peaches at the store and I was so disappointed. My first bite was unexplainable. Damn, it didn't taste like anything. There was no juice and it was dry and flavorless. I thought to myself, what is this garbage? It sure looked like a peach on the outside, but the inside was beyond horrible. I ate it anyway and placed the other four peaches into my fruit bowl. The next day I decided to eat another peach hoping the first one was bad. When I went to my fruit bowl, what I found amazed me. My four peaches were a moldy mess. Ahhhh !!!! I normally don't get angry, but on this day, I was pissed. What the hell did I buy? I spent six dollars for a bowl of mold!!! So I tossed the mold into the trash and washed my bowl. A couple weeks later, I was stupid enough to buy some more peaches just to see if I bought a bad batch. I purchased three peaches from a different store this time in the hopes of finally experiencing the pleasure of this delightful fruit. Guess what happened next. That's right. The same result once more. Yuck !!! What has happened to the goodness of our food? Food sure isn't what it used to be.

Maybe you have you noticed this too. It seems the taste of our food has disappeared. The corporate food machine has let quality fall by the waste side in the sake of quantity and profits. Therefore, the food industry has to mask these taste deficiencies with salt and sugar. Everything we eat is either too salty or too sweet. All processed food uses this formula to great success. Over the years, people have become more and more addicted to salt and sugar. Recently at a store, a random lady saw me eyeing a candy bar, which was next to some salted peanuts. She said to me, " Whatcha craving? I'm craving salt right now." I told her I was craving sweet. She said her craving the previous day was also sweet. If you think about it, these tastes are the only tastes we crave. So what good is having natural flavor if our only craving is salt or sugar? This mentality plays right into the hands of the food industry. Let's feed the masses with food like substances laden with salt and sugar because we know it is very addictive.

Have you ever seen the Sponge Bob episode where Mr. Crabs sales the Crusty Crab restaurant to a big corporation? This particular cartoon episode brought me to the realization that what we eat is just smoke and mirrors. Anyway, in this episode, this corporation sets up an assembly line to make their own version of crabby patty sandwiches. It began with a conveyor line with a big hopper of pink goop. The goop was then formed into something that resembled a patty. The goop was then spray painted brown to look like it was cooked. Afterward, dark brown lines were painted on to resemble grill marks. This concoction was conveyed into a revolving pizza oven and assembled afterward with lettuce, tomato, and a bun. It sure looked like a crabby patty sandwich, but what was it? A bunch of goop made to imitate something edible. This episode left a lasting impression in my brain. What are we actually eating anymore?

Another lasting impression is a story about one of the families at a school I once owned. This family decided to travel to Europe for 3 months. They started in Ireland and traveled all the way to Greece by land. In Great Britain, they ate the typical western diet similar to what we eat in the United States. There were fast food drive-thru's and the items in the markets appeared to be very similar to the food in the United States, except much higher priced. After they left Great Britain, this is where the food culture really changed. In France, the food was freshly made and the ingredients were produced by local farmers. The fast food joints didn't exist, except in Paris. These drive-thru restaurants probably existed to cater to the British and American tourists. As the family traveled to each country, fresh food was part of every culture. In Spain, Italy, and Germany, the food was locally grown and best of all, organic. This family said they had never experienced these flavors in the United States. If you wanted a tomato, you bought your tomato from Giuseppe the farmer. If you wanted chicken, you bought it from Diego the rancher. It was very similar to how I grew up in Central California. After two months of these wonderful culinary experiences, this family started to go through sugar and salt withdrawals. They searched and searched for some fast food to eat, but none could be found. They shortened their trip by two weeks because they couldn't handle eating great healthy food anymore. When they arrived back in Los Angeles and left customs, their first hurried stop was to Taco Bell. The whole family became extremely ill eating the Taco Bell food for the next three days. Shortly after arriving back, they noticed how much less energy they had and how much better they felt overall during their trip to Europe. The parents had lost weight on their trip but regained it all back. Soon afterward, their son became a behavioral problem and the other children began to struggle in school. Sadly, this family stayed on their American diet and never went back to this healthy lifestyle.

This story should raise some eyebrows and make you wonder if our food is actually food. For instance, let's talk about artificial colorings. Many of these colorings are derived from the petroleum industry. Yes, that means the same oil used in your cars is used in our food. Many of these colorings have been linked to several health issues from ADHD and genetic abnormalities to cancer. Why are we eating motor oil? This question needs to be addressed by our government. They have allowed the chemical companies to control the use of harmful additives in our food supply. The British government and the European Union have outlawed the use of color additives in their foods. For the sake of the mighty dollar, I guess our government believes natural colored M & M's won't sell compared to the brightly colored versions. By all costs, try to avoid artificially colored products, such as gummy foods, breakfast cereals, and fruit flavored snacks. Many of these products use petroleum-based colorants.

Have you ever noticed the beautiful pink color of salmon, which is not like any other fish in the market? The diet of wild salmon consists of crustaceans, which produce a chemical called Astaxanthin. This chemical adds this wonderful color to their meat. Since 90% of all salmon are now farm raised, the fish producers add a synthetic version of Astaxanthin to their feed to replicate this color. While natural Astaxanthin is the most powerful anti-oxidant known, the synthetic version is derived from coal tar and is very toxic. Not only are people being poisoned by mercury and radiation while eating these fish, now the farmers are poisoning the population with coal tar as well. Much of the salmon raised today is of the GMO variety, which is still under investigation regarding health safety. Maybe you should think twice before you choose sushi for dinner.

Because everyone's life matters, I hope someday soon, some of the food producers will take a step backward and supply the world with quality, unadulterated food once again. It has been proven that the masses can be fed with organic food. The media makes excuses for our tainted food supply because of overpopulation and again people are either gullible or ignorant. Our mindless society allows this exploitation to exist. Isn't it healthy to question why so many kids get autism and why our cancer rates have skyrocketed? Most of the population believes the media's propaganda as fact until tragedy strikes on a personal level. Even then, some people accept it as a natural progression and never question the cause. They depend on others to fulfill their curiosity void and accept their words as gospel. The media has perfected this. "If I heard it on the news, if must be true" is a common response for some of these individuals. Isn't this mentality similar to my goat urine story in the preface of this book?

Ultimately, refuse to trust what you hear and only trust yourself. You can listen to opinions and alternate beliefs to help form your outlook, but keep an open mind and question everything you are told. This is especially true when it comes to profits. Do you think the used car salesman will tell you the car you're looking at is held together with bubble gum and super glue? When it comes to his wallet, he will try to convince you this is the perfect car for you. The problem lies with the industries with deep pockets, like the medical industry and the food suppliers. They usually pay other firms to promote their exploits. As these people try to convince you that something is good, so is the likelihood of you buying into their false truths. Don't be a victim.

CHAPTER 15:
You Should Know Chapter

THIS FINAL CHAPTER IS dedicated to the cures and suppressed truths being withheld from the general public. Many of these items have been scattered throughout this book, so I decided to list them all in one chapter for reference purposes. Although this chapter may not cover all your questions, hopefully, it will be a guide to some of the answers. The main premise of this book is to expand your knowledge and increase your desire to become healthier. As I grew up in a money driven world (my grandfather was a banker and real estate broker), I also identified success with personal possessions and how much money was in the bank. When my school collapsed, I was left with the greatest form of wealth possible, my health. All of a sudden, money didn't matter. I was happy, healthy and dead broke. This is the beauty of this book. Health is what truly matters. Now it's time to squish the "for profit" people and take back what has been suppressed for so long. Let's start with the biggest cover-up of them all.

Cancer was originally an autoimmune disease, which was genetically mutated into a viral illness in the 1950's. The pharmaceutical companies ignored the root cause of cancer discovered by Nobel Prize winner Dr. Otto Warburg in 1931. They thought cancer could be cured by the same means as a virus. The labs took living cancer cells and included them into the polio vaccines. These vaccines were given to about 100 million people in the United States and countless others worldwide between 1955 and 1963. Although early research on hamsters indicated a strong increase in cancer tumors, the pharmaceutical companies claimed to accidently add this so called monkey virus to all their polio vaccinations. Does this smell right to you? Anyway, this vaccine is the main cause of a variety of cancers never before experienced by humans, such as certain lung, bone, brain and lymphatic cancers plus a host of others. The government denied this catastrophe from ever occurring until the Center for Disease Control finally admitted to these facts in 2007. If you or one of your parents or grandparents had one of these tainted vaccinations, you are also infected. This virus is passed on from generation to generation. If you are of Danish or Swedish decent, you were probably also subjected to this virus. Two recent discoveries indicate these vaccines are responsible for HPV (a sexually transmitted cancer) and leukemia.

In 1911, a pathologist named Peyton Rous discovered a virus could be the cause of all cancers. A farmer brought him a chicken with a large cancerous tumor on its breast. He successfully passed this cancer on to other uninfected chickens from the original tumor. The medical industry thought his theory had no validity so he stopped doing cancer research until the 1930's. Later, when science began to revisit his research, it was discovered he was correct, in some ways. He received the Nobel Prize for medicine in 1966, some 55 years after his discovery.

Dr. Otto Warberg was the first to discover cancer thrived in a low oxygen environment. If the oxygen levels dropped below 35% for any given cell, the likelihood of contracting cancer within 48 hours is highly likely. Dr. Warberg also found that having low oxygen levels within the cells increased their acidity. His research also indicated that all cancer cells are anaerobic (live without oxygen) by nature. By sending high doses of oxygen to the cells, cancer will die in this highly alkaline environment. His research became the first mainstream treatment and means of cancer prevention. Remember, this discovery was made in 1931.

In 1929, an inventor, pathologist, and microbiologist named Dr. Royal Rife invented the first and only electron microscope which made it possible to observe living microorganisms, such as bacteria and viruses. The optics were made in Germany by the famous lens manufacturer Carl Zeiss. For the first time, Dr. Rife was able to see these living creatures and through the use of a movie camera, make films of these pathogens to show the science community their appearance. By being able to observe these creatures for the first time, he wondered how they would react if they were subjected to different sound frequencies. Being an inventor, he designed a frequency generator which could be adjusted to different sound waves. He knew everything could be destroyed at a certain frequency, similar to the opera singer breaking a glass with her voice. He embarked on this journey to analyze what frequencies could be utilized to destroy these microorganisms. He recorded all the data in which 2,000 different organisms were destroyed. Dr. Rife then decided to try the same technique via a plasma tube on patients with different diseases, such as tuberculosis, hepatitis, flu, common cold, and cancer. What he found out was astounding. The frequency generator would kill the microorganisms associated with these illnesses without doing any harm to the patients. The first true cancer cure was discovered through his research in 1931.

In the same year that this remarkable discovery was first published, he and the University of Southern California opened a cancer clinic in Pasadena, California to treat such diseases. The clinic had a success rate for cancer of 90% with this new found technology. From 1931 to 1934, the clinic operated without problems or issues. When the clinic started to gain notoriety as a successful treatment for all viral and bacterial based illnesses, the American Medical Association launched an all-out war to discredit the work of this clinic. Since this new technology didn't require surgery or a bunch of expensive drugs, the AMA didn't want this cure to exist. Big Medicine attacked this new technology through the court system, claiming is was quackery. New legislation was enacted to forbid this treatment from ever being used and the clinic was ordered to close with all its equipment to be destroyed. In June of 1937, the clinic was shut down permanently. This revolutionary cure was destroyed because the medical industry saw the end of their existence. Fortunately, some of the equipment was shipped to other locations and all the research notes were preserved by Dr. Rife.

I met an ex-doctor, whose license was revoked for curing people with this wonderful device. His clinic was shut down and destroyed with sledgehammers. Every employee at the clinic, during the time of the seizure, was arrested and stripped of their medical licenses. Many of the doctors served in prison for breaking the curing law. This ex-doctor escaped prosecution because he was on vacation at the time of the seizure. The wellness center operated for three years with over 2,000 patients being cured. Their 90% success rate was based on all forms of cancer, including the hardest to cure, bone cancer. This ex-doctor is now in hiding to avoid serving prison time. He told me the frequency generator is the only known cure for all types of cancer. The 10% of the patients who died were the people who had given up hope and lost their will to live. These are the people who believe there is no cure and have been brainwashed by our media. He explained to me if a person has a strong will to live, the frequency generator would cure them. His story gave me the inspiration to write this chapter. The only reason I met this man was because a former patient of his told me he was a miracle worker who cured her of stage 4 breast and bone cancer. He was very hesitant to talk until I explained I was writing a book for the sake of humanity. He cried during our interview. His passion for helping others was squished by Big Medicine for the sake of profits. I could see he was a shell of his former self, like many of the people I write about in this book. Big Medicine demoralized their love for helping others, just like this ex-doctor.

A remarkable German/Jewish physician named Dr. Max Gerson suffered from severe migrate headaches while in college. He decided to try to relieve his headaches through diet. He formulated a juice and soup diet using only organic produce, which eliminated all dairy and meat products. Through his observations, he discovered his headaches were caused by animal toxins not being eliminated by an unhealthy liver. He discovered that by using coffee enemas, the caffeine would stimulate the bile ducts in the intestines and clear out any unwanted toxins that may be stored in the liver. Almost immediately, his headaches were eliminated and they never came back.

Later as a licensed physician, one of his patients he was treating for migraines noticed that their skin tuberculosis had also been cured. At this time, there was no known cure for the highly infectious bacterial condition. This caught the attention of world-renowned surgeon Ferdinand Sauerbruch. He partnered up with Dr. Gerson to do a clinical study on the effects of his therapy in regards to skin tuberculosis. The results were astounding. Out of the 460 patients in the study, 456 were cured of this horrible illness. Soon after, Dr. Gerson became a household name in Europe for his remarkable cure.

In 1938, Dr. Gerson fled Germany to avoid the holocaust and migrated to the United States. He passed his bar exam and opened an office in Manhattan, New York. Soon after opening his office, a patient came to him with gall bladder and stomach cancer. She first heard of him in Europe and thought he could cure her condition. Initially, Dr. Gerson refused to treat her because of the political scrutiny he could face if she happened to be cured. After a tremendous amount of persuasion by his patient, he privately cured her of cancer using his protocol. Unable to live with this incredible discovery, he decided to treat only the patient's other doctors left to die. His success rate was remarkable for these terminally ill individuals. He reported a 38% survival rate for all cancer patients to live a full lifetime, while with today's medicine the survival rate is only 24% to live for 5 years and 2.1% to fulfill a normal lifespan.

In 1946, President Harry Truman decided to wage a war of cancer. He vowed to allocate two billion dollars to this fight with a 100 million dollars going to the establishment with the best cure and continued research. Dr. Gerson was asked to speak in front of a senate committee about his wonderful cure. He spent two days speaking in this hearing along with many of his cured patients praising this healthy treatment. As a result, ABC news publicly reported that a cure had been found for cancer. Unfortunately, four of the senators on this committee were also medical doctors and his cure was abolished to prevent this protocol from ever being implemented in the United States. Once again, Big Medicine wiped out another tremendous cancer cure. The money allocated for cancer research never came to fruition and the ABC reporter, who reported this wonderful news to the nation, was fired and discredited. He was never allowed to work in the news field ever again. A retraction to his story was announced and Dr. Gerson's protocol was reported to be a hoax. Dr. Gerson moved to San Diego, California when his medical license was revoked in the state of New York. For the next 20 years, Dr. Gerson operated his own cancer clinic in Tijuana, Mexico, since laws were enacted to prevent his cure from being used in the United States. In 1958, he published a book on his protocol with much scrutiny from the medical establishment. He was poisoned to death the following year by a medical insider.

His daughter currently has continued her father's work and has established 360 clinics worldwide for this cancer treatment. The clinics have cured several members of the British royal family and the wife of Nobel Prize winner Dr. Albert Schweitzer of her lung tuberculosis and his diabetes. Dr. Schweitzer remained Dr. Gerson's leading advocate and gave his eulogy at his funeral. Our war on cancer is not about curing this disease; it's about killing the un-patentable and unprofitable cures. If Big Medicine can't have their hands on the treatment, the treatment will not exist. You can see how far they'll go to protect this money making machine.

As previously mentioned in chapter 7, Dr. Johanna Budwig was a 6 time Nobel Prize nominee and her protocol has an over 90% success rate for curing all forms of cancers. As well, this protocol is also a cure for 50 other illnesses. Her clinic is still operational and curing people of such conditions. Today, the Budwig Protocol is the most successful cure for stage 4 cancer. In Germany, she was able to operate without the fear of the political corruptness.

In the United States, the American Cancer Society is still trying to raise money to find the cure. However, the cure will never be applied because the law specifies it is illegal to cure, only to treat the disease. How much more contradictory can a country become? The ACS will keep trying to defraud the American public until they find a new treatment that can be patented. The ignorant and gullible are the people feeding this corrupt system.

One the greatest discovery in cancer treatments and a cure for herpes is associated with a natural industrial solvent called Dimethyl Sulfoxide or DMSO for short. This by-product of the tree industries was first discovered in 1866, however, its first medical use didn't appear until 1961. DMSO is easily absorbed through the skin and had been used for many different ailments. This extraordinary anti-inflammatory and anti-oxidant solvent has been tested in 125 countries for its medical properties. This compound has been discredited in the United States by the FDA since 1963 because a woman had died from an allergic reaction to an unknown substance while conducting the clinical trials. The FDA immediately (without investigation) blamed DMSO as the culprit and shut down all trials. It was banned for human use in 1967, except for a patented drug for a bladder condition. With all the clinical trials performed in the other countries on this miracle solvent, no other person has died from its use. What is astounding is DMSO is available to treat your pets and animals of a wide variety of ailments. The race horse industry uses this solvent for sprains and strains with immediate results. This compound works just as well on humans. However, it can cause some redness to the skin.

The most remarkable discovery regarding DMSO was in the treatment of cancer. The alternative cancer industry calls it the magic bullet to cure cancer. DMSO opens the pores of the cancer cells to allow the penetration other cancer eliminating compounds. Think of DMSO as a Trojan horse for the cure. When DMSO enters the blood stream, it targets only the cancer cells to become more responsive. There are several different cancer protocols which use DMSO as its main ingredient. For instance, a doctor in Atlanta, Georgia decided to do some experimenting with this compound. Being a western medical doctor and relying on chemo, radiation, and surgeries as his only legal options for treatment, he decided to give his patients DMSO before their radiation treatments. What he found was remarkable. DMSO seemed to only target the cancer cells and actually protected the normal cells from damage caused by the radiation. He also discovered that he could reduce the radiation levels to 1/10 of the normal strength with tremendous success. He was actually curing people with radiation and not killing the whole body, like traditional radiation treatments. The medical industry found out about his methods and promptly shutting down his clinic and stripped him of his license. Again, curing patients is illegal in the United States.

If DMSO is used with any other known cancer killers like vitamins C and D3, insulin, ozonated water, colloidal silver and chemotherapy drugs, the success rate is remarkable. Research has shown that DMSO can also dissolve blood clots after having a stroke, which will reduce the likelihood of brain damage. So why is DMSO banned for human use? The reason is a tub of this gel costs $13.95 at your local animal feed store. When the average cost is two million dollars per cancer patient until death and hundreds of thousands to treat a stroke, $13.95 is just not profitable enough for Big Medicine.

I believe the American Medical Association's motto should be "Profits over Humanity". Do you believe the media when they promote the United States as having the best healthcare system in the world? If you happen to be one of those ignorant or gullible people, I have little sympathy for your condition. I do believe the US had the most profitable and best diagnostic medical system. By diagnosing non-existent illnesses, such as diabetes for non-diabetics, this system will keep flourishing with record profits for a very long time. This is just one example of this corrupt system.

A famous Italian surgeon named Dr. Tullio Simoncini became very curious why cancer tumors were white, instead of red in color. He knew cancer was very resilient and would create its own circulatory system to insure its survival, so he figured that cancer tumors should be red. So one day he decided to do a composition test on a cancer tumor. What the lab found out was amazing. The tumor was white because a great portion of its composition was made of a fungus. This fungus called Candida Albicans is formed from the consumption of yeast. Candida Albicans is normally a healthy bacteria used to break down foods in the digestive tract. What Dr. Simoncini discovered is if our immune system is compromised, this bacteria can leave the gut and aid in the formation of cancer tumors. Being a western medical doctor, he thought prescription anti-bacterial medications would help kill the cancer cells. What he discovered was the cancer cells mutated every couple of days, so the medications were ineffective. He then started to research to find what the best antibacterial and antifungal substance known to humankind. What he discovered was baking soda was extremely effective at killing household germs and it's non-toxic to humans in small quantities. Dr. Simoncini first tried to have his patients take baking soda orally, which produced mixed results. One day, Dr. Simoncini was installing a port into a patient for their radiation treatments when he realized he could probably use baking soda instead of the radiation. He tried this method with this patient and saw instant results. The cancer tumor had disappeared. That's when he realized that his new treatment would be successful. He started to prescribed douches to his female patients who had cancer of the uterus and cervical cancer. The combination of distilled water with 2 tablespoons of baking soda had a tremendous success rate.

   He began using these techniques in his normal practice until the medical establishment discovered his cure. He was attacked as a fraud and was publicly scrutinized and ridiculed by the media. The paparazzi were dispatched to chase him down and harass him since he was already a public figure. Ultimately, he was stripped of his medical license and sent to jail for 3 years for manslaughter. He was prosecuted because one of his terminally ill patients died while doing his treatment. During the court proceedings, the judge ruled his treatment may have compromised his patient's health. Many of his cured patients testified in court on his behalf, including other medical doctors, yet the judge still ruled against him.

Dr. Simoncini claimed his cancer success rate was 90% for non-terminal patients and 50% for terminally ill patients. He later wrote a book after his conviction entitled *Cancer is a Fungus: A Revolution in Tumor Therapy*. The University of Arizona received a two million dollar grant to investigate the use of baking soda as an alternative cancer treatment. The research showed by using baking soda orally, it would reduce or eliminated several cancers from spreading. The only drawback found was over time, baking soda caused some organ damage resulting from the overabundance of sodium in the body. It is recommended to take breaks using this protocol. The recommended interval is 3 months of treatment with a one month break between cycles.

Although there is much speculation on how baking soda kills cancer, its effectiveness can't be denied. Many experts believe baking soda attacks the microbes inside the cancer cells. Others believe the alkalinity associated with this product kills cancer, while Dr. Simoncini believes baking soda kills the fungus associated with cancer, which makes it so effective. I personally believe it is a combination of all of the above. Any way you look at it, baking soda is a tremendous tool and it should be used for several health-related reasons. From a non-fluoride alternative toothpaste to regulating pH levels to making vitamin C much more effective, baking soda should be a staple of everyone's diet.

From 1900 to 1930, electro-medicine was being taught in all medical schools and was the most effective way of ridding the body of all known pathogens. Even Sears and Robuck sold these devices to the general public through their catalogs. When the pharmaceutical companies took over the medical universities, the American Medical Association and Federal

Drug Administration outlawed the use of these electro-medicine devices because of its lack of profitability. They enacted laws against the use of such devices unless approved by their establishments. The effectiveness of these devices is unparalleled to any of the medications used today. I feel this decision by our government to choose profits over humanity has caused the demise of our health care system.

Although electro-medicine has been around since the turn of the 20th century, Dr. Bob Beck is considered the godfather and leading advocate of reinstituting electro-medicine back into mainstream medical practices. Dr. Beck was physicist, inventor and an innovator of such devices. His most recognizable invention was the electronic flash for cameras. Over the years, Dr. Beck re-examined many of the patents used in the field of electromedicine from the early 1900's and re-engineered these devices using modern electronics. He funded his own testing and created a protocol to cure all illnesses called the Beck Protocol. It is a four-step series of different treatments to achieve great health and to relieve all the symptoms of pre-existing illnesses.

The first and most important step in this protocol is the use of an electrical shock blood purifier. Dr. Beck's research discovered if blood was hit with a small electrical charge in a pulsating fashion, the electricity would kill all living organisms in the blood over several months. Later studies also showed that the living organisms which remained alive after the use of the blood purifier could not replicate when electrified, which include viruses, bacteria, fungus, microbes, and parasites.

Most humans carry between 1 1/2 pounds to 3 pounds of living organisms at any given time. Eventually, through this treatment, these organisms will die and enable the immune system to become supercharged. Typically, our immune system is continually fighting these living creatures throughout our lifetime. This protocol rids our bodies of these invaders associated with such illnesses as cancer, HIV, the flu and any other pathogen based conditions.

Based on a self-funded study, Dr. Beck found the blood purifier could kill the HIV virus in as little as two weeks and also halt the spread of cancer. He presented this study to the AMA and was promptly discredited because their flawed testing painted a different picture. It has since been proven the testing by the AMA should have been discredited instead. A severe flaw was detected in their procedure. The AMA is still backing their inaccurate results.

Dr. Beck's blood purifier is a small electrolysis device, which was intended for daily use. This device can be constructed for around $8 at Radio Shack. The AMA's profit machine wouldn't allow such a device to exist based on the 2017 drug prices of $18,300 per year for HIV treatment. As a cure for many deadly illnesses, this device would have taken away billions of dollars from Big Medicine if it had continued to sell on the open market.

The second phase of the protocol was created to compliment the blood purifier. Since other pathogens hide in our lymph system, stomach, liver, dental work and other organs, Dr. Beck discovered a way to release these creatures into our blood stream to be destroyed by the blood purifier. Since all organisms need to be removed to supercharge our immune system, Dr. Beck found by introducing magnetic pulses to these body parts, the organisms would come out of hiding. It's like shaking the dog house to make your dog come out. Once the creatures are released, the blood purifier would neutralize them with electricity. This device can easily be made for about $40 from parts found at your local yard sale/swap meet/flea market and electronics store.

Dr. Beck often used his inventions on himself to ensure their safety. What he discovered was this device could regrow hair. He was once balding and by using the magnetic pulser, his hair regrew as fine baby hair and in its original color. This amazing discovery stunned Bob more than any of his other inventions since he had some personal insecurity regarding his hair loss.

The third phase of the protocol has been around for thousands of years. Up until the 1930's when the pharmaceutical companies destroyed the previous medical system, silver was considered the best anti-microbial agent ever known to humankind. What is so remarkable is silver is still the most effective pathogen killer in existence over any prescription drug. The saying "He was born with a silver spoon in his mouth" has much validity. In ancient times, silver was used to make urns to keep the water and wine away from living organisms. Research has shown the best antibiotics today kill about a dozen pathogens, while silver kills about 650. This information will become extremely valuable when the pharmaceutical companies unleash their man-made viruses on the general public. These viruses will be released to corner the market on new drugs and create population control. I hope this is a reality check for some since this is happening right in front of our faces. These companies even have the gall to announce their intentions to the general public. However, most people won't heed their warnings. They will go to their doctors and get the latest antibiotic to hopefully keep themselves alive.

The best form of silver for medical purposes is a liquid called colloidal silver. This product is basically distilled water with tiny particles of silver infused into this water. Colloidal silver can be used orally, topically or intravenously without any side effects. By drinking 1 ounce of colloidal silver daily, most pathogens will die within the body. This is especially true for cancer cells. The anti-pathogenic properties of colloidal silver are very effective at killing the microbes within the cancer cells and returning them back to their normal state.

The most effective way to kill cancer is to hit it from all angles and with great intensity. Would a fireman try to put out a fire with a squirt gun? Of course not. Unfortunately, this is what happens to most patients. The doctors are limited to what they've learned in medical school and it just isn't enough. This is especially true with pneumonia. The fireman should have the most resources as possible to put out that fire. This is the basis of the Beck Protocol. It makes more sense to fight illness from every angle and possible way and not just using drugs put into the blood stream.

If one is to purchase colloidal silver, the price is extremely expensive. A small 4-ounce bottle can cost between $40USD to $100USD. Dr. Beck discovered a way to make colloidal silver for a few meager pennies. By attaching wires to a series of 9-volt batteries along with a couple pieces of .999 pure silver, Dr. Beck was able to produce his own colloidal silver. This very simple process can be created by almost anyone. Put distilled water into a glass container and suspend the silver pieces so half the silver is in the water and the other half is in the air. Make sure the silver pieces are not touching each other. Hook up a series of batteries to wires and alligator clips. Clamp the clips onto the silver and watch. As the silver dissipates into the water, the water will become cloudy with a silverish/blue tint. When light is no longer able to penetrate through the glass, the colloidal silver will be ready to drink. You just produced the best antibiotics known on this Earth. Your cold, flu or even your cancer will become a thing of the past with this wonderful product.

The fourth phase of the protocol is the use of ozonated water. Throughout the book, I have referenced ozonated water for many purposes. Ozonated water is basically over oxygenated water. Standard water has two atoms of hydrogen and one atom of oxygen to make H_2O. If we add another oxygen atom to water, we make hydrogen peroxide or H_2O_2. We know hydrogen peroxide is a wonderful antiseptic used for wounds and it is also very useful in restaurants to kill bacteria found in kitchens. By adding ozone gas to standard water, two extra oxygen atoms are added to the water to make H_2O_3. Unfortunately, this gas is easily expelled from the water in about 20 minutes. This incredible technology is used in Europe to sterilize their water supply. While is the United States, most of our water is sterilized with chemicals, such as chlorine. The hospitals in Germany and Russia give freshly ozonated water to all their patients throughout their stay. These hospitals also pump ozone gas into their air conditioning units to keep the whole hospital sterilized. How many times have you gone to the ER and wondered if you would contract some deadly illness while in the waiting room? In Germany and Russia, they want their citizens healthy, while is the US, the hospitals hope you contract another illness to increase their profits. I almost lost a dear friend from a staph infection she contracted while waiting for her mother in an emergency room. Dr. Beck himself coined the phrase' "A patient cured is a patient lost". He must have been thinking about the medical system in the United States when he made that statement.

By adding two extra atoms of oxygen to the water, this super antiseptic has been known to kill 100% of all the known pathogens on this planet. Not only will it kill the bad creatures living within us, it will also kill the good bacteria needed for proper digestion. A good probiotic is needed while drinking this water and colloidal silver since both compounds will kill the pathogens in our digestive system. It is recommended one should drink 4 ounces of ozonated water daily for a maintenance program and up to 32 ounces for a stage 4 cancer patient. I drink ozonated water for my pre-workout beverage with great success. The water seems to help my energy levels toward the end of my workout when all my fuel has already been spent.

Since freshly ozonated water is required, Ebay and Amazon carry such units priced from $30USD to $500USD. Many aquarium shops also carry water ozonators to purify their tanks. The small inexpensive units work perfectly fine for a family. There is no need to purchase the larger unit unless you intend to disinfect your home. If you choose to purchase a larger unit, bathing in ozonated water has significant health advantages. From killing skin cancer to acne issues, allowing your skin to be rejuvenated by these extra oxygen atoms is almost euphoric. Not only will you benefit from this added oxygen, ozonated water is also the best antiseptic known to humankind. Your skin will become 100% pathogen free, after one of these wonderful baths. Also explained in previous chapters, your produce should be washed with ozonated water to release the pesticides and to kill any pathogens lingering on the surface of your produce.

There are some disturbing side effects associated with the Beck Protocol. As mention in earlier chapters, the possibility of an individual experiencing Herxheimer Syndrome is extremely likely. The other major side effect is your body will experience skin eruptions. These eruptions could appear anywhere since your body is ridding itself of all the pathogens living within us. The dead parasites, bacteria, microbes and viruses can't all be excreted through our liver and kidneys. Since our skin is the largest organ in our body and is very effective at flushing unwanted waste, these eruptions can flair up in some very strange locations. As gross and annoying as this may be, this is very good for your health. When the Herxheimer symptoms and the eruptions stop, your body's immune system will be able to fight off every known pathogenic illness. This process may take up to 6 months to complete, but after this time, you may experience a true medical anomaly. This anomaly is called immortal blood. By ridding your body of all pathogens, your white blood cells will stay dormant because there is nothing for them to fight. This condition can create true immortality, at least from the standpoint of outside invaders trying to create havoc within us.

When Dr. Max Gerson first discovered a healthy liver was the key to health, many other doctors heeded his philosophy and expanded on his protocol. Western medicine lists too many incurable diseases which actually have cures. These cures have been blackballed by the establishment because Big Medicine hasn't found a patentable treatment for such illnesses. One of the leading remedies is a liver and gall bladder flush. With the average adult having between 300 and 1,000 gall stones interfering with the expulsion of toxins, a gallbladder and liver flush is the proper treatment to help clear this unwanted waste. Having known of an effective procedure to clean out these unwanted stones, I asked a medical doctor what was the best way to rid ourselves of these obstructions. His answer was only through surgery. I explained that there was an easier and less evasive way to relieve these stones and he became rather upset. I dropped the subject to remedy the situation. This narrow-minded doctor is part of the problem. I have wondered if some doctors actually believe what they have learned in medical school could be incorrect or misleading? I believe we are only as good as what we've been taught. If you are taught incorrect information, then the false answers become the truth. This fact has become very evident in today's medical profession.

Our liver produces a fluid called bile, which is stored in the gall bladder. Bile is used in the digestion process to break down fats. The gallbladder is attached to the small intestines through small tubes called bile ducts. When fatty foods are eaten, the intestines send a signal to the liver asking for help. The gallbladder releases bile to help digest the fatty foods. Not only does bile help with digestion, bile also is a means to flush out unwanted cholesterol and fat-soluble toxins from our liver. If the bile ducts are clogged with gallstones, the bile cannot be released properly into the intestines. This obstruction can affect the digestion of food and the expulsion of toxic matter.

The most efficient and least evasive way to rid the body of these stones is with a liver and gall bladder flush. This cleanse will require four basic ingredients, sour cherry juice, fresh grapefruit, Epsom Salts and a healthy oil like olive oil or coconut oil. The sour cherry juice contained malic acid, which softens the gallstones for better secretion. The combination of fresh grapefruit juice and Epsom salts dilates the bile ducts to prepare for the release of the stones. These ingredients also allow the liver to create an extra large amount of bile needed to expel the stones. A large amount of oil is required to release all the stored bile at once to flush out the stones. After the procedure, the stones released will float when you use the restroom. This will give you a strong indication of how effective the flush was on your liver. Some people may release a couple of small stones, while others may have hundreds. I had one client release 3 little stones floating on top of her feces, while another client told me he could not see his feces because the toilet water was covered in stones. It all depends on how well you follow the instructions and how many stones are in your gall bladder before the flush.

To start the cleanse, it is advisable to drink 8 ounces of the sour cherry juice per day for 6 days. By drinking this juice, the process will become more effective. If sour cherry juice is too expensive or too hard to locate, apple juice can be substituted instead. However, a quart of apple juice is required daily due to a lower amount of malic acid associated with apple juice compared to sour cherry juice. If possible, try to buy or make your own apple juice. The processed juice contains fewer nutrients due to the pasteurization process. If the sugar content in the apple juice is the main deterring issue, sour cherry juice is much lower in sugar. It is best to drink the juice throughout the day so your body has a continuous supply of malic acid. On the day of flush, drink the juice only in the morning. A vegetarian diet is recommended using only room temperature foods and beverages. Ice cold food and beverages tend to decrease the effectiveness of the flush because of the added stress created by the cold foods on the liver.

If you are dependent on prescription drugs, it is advisable to wean yourself off of these drugs before doing the cleanse. Most prescriptions drugs cause more damage than good to the liver so your results will be less than satisfactory. Many of these drugs can cause an adverse effect when the liver dumps all its toxins into the blood stream at the same time. When it comes to cancer medications, it's advisable to wait 6-8 months after the last drugs were taken before starting your cleanse. These drugs create a different type of gallstones. When released, these stones can cause a multitude of adverse effects on the body. It's advisable to consult a naturopathic doctor months before the cleanse to locate natural substitutions for your current medicines. The only exception is for those individuals on thyroid medications. This medication cannot be substituted or eliminated due to the life-threatening consequences that may occur if these drugs are not administered. The flush should not be scheduled on a full moon. During a full moon, the body retains more water than normal, which makes the cleanse less effective. To avoid becomes nauseated during the flush, it is recommended to do a thorough colon cleanse on the day of the treatment. Most ill effects associated with this flush are caused by the improper elimination of the toxin in the bowels prior to the cleanse. The best colon cleanse is a hydro colonic treatment before the flush. This therapy will eliminate 85% of all the accumulated fecal matter in the colon. If this therapy is an impossibility, a simple water enema will suffice. Eating a vegetarian diet a week leading up to the flush will help eliminate the extra toxins inside the digestive system. Avoid any fatty foods during this week. Since bile is used to aid the digestion of fat, eating fatty foods will decrease the amount of bile needed for a proper flush. If your body has not stored enough bile prior the flush, you may also become very ill.

On the day of the flush, do not eat or drink anything except for water after 1:30 pm. By eating or drinking before the flush, this action will severely hinder its effectiveness. Do not drink water for 10-15 minutes after drinking the Epsom salts solution. This will hinder the effectiveness of the flush as well. At 6:00 pm, add 4 tablespoons of Epsom salts to 24 ounces of water. At this time, drink 1/4 of the solution. If the bitter taste is too difficult to handle, you can add a little lemon juice to the mixture to improve the taste. Make sure your grapefruit is at room temperature at this time. The grapefruit will be used in the next couple of hours. At 8:00 pm, drink another 6 ounces of the mixture. By 9:30 pm, a bowel movement should have occurred unless you properly cleansed your colon. If you didn't do a colon cleanse, it is recommended to perform a water enema at this time to make sure the bile ducts will remain open and unclogged for the next phase of the cleanse. At 9:45 pm, squeeze your grapefruit until you make 6 ounces of juice. Add 4 ounces of oil to the grapefruit juice into a glass container with a lid. Shake the mixture until the contents are thorough combined. At 10:00 pm, drink this mixture while standing. It is critical that you stand while drinking this concoction. Try to finish the mixture within 5 minutes and immediately lay down on your back. Get a couple of pillows to prop your head up. Your head must maintain the same level as your abdomen. Remain still in this position for 20 minutes and use your brain to concentrate on your liver. The brain can help this process tremendously. Imagine your body releasing these stones. As explained in an earlier chapter, the mind can heal you or kill you. Do not drink water for 2 hours after drinking the oil solution. The water will make the flush less effective. The first 20 minutes is extremely critical in this process. After the first 20 minutes, you may move into your normal sleeping position, except do not sleep on your stomach. If you feel like having a bowel movement, please do so. You may see some of the stones released in the toilet at this time. At 6-6:30 the next morning, drink a glass of warm water and another 6 ounces of the Epsom salts mixture. If you feel low on energy, go back to bed. If possible, try to remain upright for the next two hours. At 8-8:30 am, drink the last of the Epsom salts mixture. At 10-10:30 am, you may drink a small glass of fruit juice. A half an hour later, you may eat a piece or two of fruit. Around 12:00 pm, you are permitted to eat a light vegetarian meal. For the next 2-3 days, eat light meals since your body just completed a tremendous cleansing procedure.

According to the historical record, apple cider vinegar first came into existence 7,000 years ago. Since its invention, this vinegar has been used as a remedy for many illnesses throughout time. From digestive issues to helping relieve varicose veins, apple cider vinegar is one of the two greatest natural healers known to exist. The best form of this vinegar is the unfiltered variety with the mother. This cloudy vinegar contained living bacteria from the yeast used in the fermentation process. This bacteria is essential for many of the listed remedies below. Let's break down some of the many cures and remedies associated with this gift of nature.

There are many uses for apple cider vinegar related to digestive health. As explained in the previous paragraph, this vinegar contains bacteria. This bacteria is a natural probiotic needed to break down and digest our foods. If you experience constipation issues, apple cider vinegar may be a less evasive remedy for your condition.

If you are experiencing heartburn, this vinegar may also be a wonderful solution for your condition. The root cause of heartburn is weak stomach acid. Since this product is extremely acidic, this vinegar combines with the existing stomach acid to create a more powerful acid needed to break down our foods during digestion. By increasing the strength of your stomach acid, your body won't need to over produce to compensate for the weak acid already in our stomach.

When it comes to common viral ailments like sore throats and colds, apple cider vinegar is a wonderful alternative for many of the over the counter medicines. Since apple cider vinegar has powerful anti-pathogenic properties, many of these illnesses can be warded off by this incredible product. Not only is apple cider vinegar a natural antibiotic, it is full of important antioxidants and vitamins to supercharge your immune system to rid yourself of these unwanted illnesses.

Apple cider vinegar has many uses related to our skin, hair, and nails. Since this vinegar has powerful anti-pathogenic properties, this product has been known to relieve symptoms of nail fungus, eczema, varicose veins, and acne, when used topically.

When applied to the hair in a diluted solution, this product has been known to rid the hair follicles of the wax buildup caused by chemical based shampoos and conditioners. This solution will leave your hair shiny and healthy. Some individuals have experienced hair growth as a result of this solution. When taken topically and internally, this solution may cure male pattern baldness in some individuals. Many have seen remarkable results after 3 months of continuous use.

Along with citrus fruits, apple cider vinegar is a tremendous pH balancing product. Even though this vinegar is acidic, it actually absorbs other acids within our bodies for elimination. This makes apple cider vinegar an excellent cancer fighter and can relieve many of the symptoms associated with extremely high acids levels such as gout.

Apple cider vinegar is a wonderful blood purifier and liver detoxifier which help support many of the internal glands and organs explained in chapter 1. Going back to its anti-pathogenic properties, this vinegar can fend off many of the microbes and parasites living within our body. This pathogen fighter is also beneficial to the health of our lymph system. Since many of these living creatures hide within these areas, apple cider vinegar can eliminate these critters and release the toxins stored within our body.

Many conditions caused by inflammation, such as arthritis, can be relieved by apple cider vinegar. When added to other anti-inflammatory compounds, such as cactus and a few amino acids like L-Methionine, this product can relieve much of the swelling in the joints for tremendous relief.

Apple cider vinegar contains a compound called acetic acid. This incredible acid is only found in the apple cider vinegar which contains the mother. This incredible acid is wonderful for diabetics, people with high cholesterol and individuals trying to lose weight. For diabetics, this acid blocks some of the starch from being digested. Since starch is a form of sugar, this acid will lower your blood sugar. Another wonderful effect of acetic acid is it blocks the cravings to eat sugar. This is especially important to both people trying to lose weight as well as diabetics. If these individuals consume less sugar based foods, this allows their need for insulin to decrease. For weight loss, acetic acid is one of the best natural fat burners, along with berries and citrus fruits. For people with cholesterol issues, apple cider vinegar tends to lower their LDL or bad cholesterol, yet increase their HDL or good cholesterol at the same time. When combined with niacin, this mixture can control your cholesterol levels better than any medication prescribed by your doctor and it's all natural.

For those on blood-thinning medications, such as aspirin therapy, the acetic acid in apple cider vinegar is just as effective as many of these medicines and without the serious side effects associated with these drugs.

Can you understand why I feel apple cider vinegar is one of the greatest tools ever discovered for the greater good of humankind? It can even replace all your cleaning products in your house. Maybe it's time to throw out all those chemical based compounds and let nature take care of your dirty work instead.

I bet you're wondering what the second greatest natural healer could be since the first one was so tremendous. The second natural remedy for most illnesses is coconut oil. As explained briefly is chapter 5, you will see why I believe coconut trees exist on small islands throughout this planet. Let's take a look at the second wonder of the nutritional world.

In the Philippines, the coconut tree is referred to as the "Tree of Life" and in Malaysia, it is known as the "Tree of a Thousand Uses". Any way you look at it, these cultures knew what they were saying. The coconut holds a special place among the greatest creations on Earth.

Like apple cider vinegar, coconut oil is very useful for the skin health. This oil has proven to smooth out wrinkles and reduce age spots. It works as a natural moisturizer and also exhibits anti-pathogenic properties, similar to apple cider vinegar. Coconut oil can also help relieve flaking associated with such skin conditions as eczema, psoriasis, dermatitis and dandruff. This oil can be used as a tanning oil and relieve burns by hydrating the affected area. As an antiseptic, coconut oil works well to kill any germs which can cause infection. If used topically on the area with cellulite, coconut oil can smooth out the fat under the skin for a more pleasant appearance.

Coconut oil has also been proven to help relieve many of the symptoms associated with Alzheimer's disease. This wonderful oil is basically the perfect brain food. Since coconut oil is digested differently than other oils, it effectively supplies the brain with all its critical nutrients and has been proven to decrease memory loss and reverse some of the effects of this horrible disease.

Like apple cider vinegar, coconut oil is also wonderful for diabetics. This oil has been proven to balance blood sugar by increasing the insulin response by the pancreas, similar to ingesting protein. This makes this oil very desirable to diabetics while cooking carb based foods.

Coconut oil works very effectively on several digestive issues. This oil has been proven to help individuals affected by Leaky Gut Syndrome. The anti-pathogenic properties of this amazing oil can also rid the body of many other conditions such as yeast infections, cancer microbes, and fungi. Coconut oil also contains necessary gut bacteria essential for the proper digestion of foods, similar to probiotics.

Many other conditions coconut oil can remedy are kidney infections, arthritis pain, liver detoxifying, can halt osteoporosis, lower bad cholesterol and balance the hormones, just to name a few. Coconut oil is also a tremendous energy booster and is a natural fat burner. This oil can also boost the immune system, similar to taking an anti-oxidant supplements.

If you decide not to heed the other information in this book except for the use of apple cider vinegar and coconut oil, your quality of life will improve considerably. This shows the power of these two incredible products in regards to treating many of the ailments associated with today's society.

I hope this chapter enlightens you on some of the natural cures and remedies which the health care system has tried to repress. If we use some of the preventive measures, our body will flourish and remain healthy well into our twilight years. Unfortunately, humans possess too many self-destructive tendencies to fully embrace all the tools set forth in this chapter. Are you one of the rare individuals who can? It takes work and determination to achieve great health. Since we only have one chance on this planet, why not try.

Conclusion

I HOPE READING THIS book has helped to enlighten us humans on the pitfalls we have to overcome to achieve true health. It's a hard path to follow, but the reward is to achieve a high quality of life for a very long time. Don't we owe it to ourselves to be healthy? When I see people my age struggle to do everyday tasks, it really hits me where it hurts, in my heart. The gullible, ignorant and less fortunate are the people I see laboring throughout their lives. By opening up our mind to new ideas and being aware of your surroundings, much of these problems can be prevented. For the unfortunate, there are solutions. When I lost everything, I found ways to eat and stay healthy. The dollar stores have a bunch of great healthy foods if you know what to look for. Again, educate yourself and your problems will become your solutions.

The medical and food industries are out of control and the government is allowing this to happen. People have become money bags to this corporate greed and our lives hang in the balance. I sometimes feel we are just cattle being herded to the slaughterhouse just like cows. We are given drugs and poor food to kill us a little earlier than we should die. They prey on our human nature to accept or ignore the incorrect information we are being fed on a daily basis. This misinformation leads us to believe the unthinkable. People who are free thinkers are often labeled as crazy by society due to a form of brainwashing and cast away from our regular population. "Oh, that person is just crazy because she thinks extraterrestrials exist" is a prime example. A free thinker will question life on other planets and the origin of our existence. Others will follow their religious beliefs as gospel and many will believe there is no other way. Since the majority of people follow the established norm, this makes us the prey for others to dictate our lives. I hope this book enlightened you to question what is really being fed to us, both physically and mentally.

It is time for a world figure to stand up and fight this system for the betterment of humanity. Even as powerful as the pharmaceutical companies have become, it's time for them to take a back seat in the sake of our survival. We are fed a bunch of lies making drugs appear to be healthy. DRUGS ARE NOT HEALTH FOOD!!! Drugs and chemicals cause the majority of the medical issues we experience today. As explained throughout this book, there is a natural cure for almost every disease and drugs do not cure anything. The only thing drugs do is make a lot of money for the government and the medical industry. If you happen to use the tools in chapter 15, you may never need any of their adult candy again. Drugs do nothing for you except kill you faster. Nature has given us everything we need to stay healthy and to prosper. It is time to go back to nature.

Thank you for purchasing this book. While on this wonderful journey, I hope you accept a small part of me as your own. All I can do is hope you embrace these words and make improvements in your life. If you feel compelled to share this book or any of this information with others, please do so. This book was intended to be an awakening. If every person who comes in contact with these pages receives a small gift of life, my job as a writer has been accomplished. Please enjoy a long and healthy life, with as much quality as a person can expect. I wrote this book for you.

Index

3

3 Mile Island, 101

A

AARP, 106
abdomen, 33, 134
absorbic acid, 80
acetic acid, 136, 137
acidic, 35, 44, 55, 74, 75, 76, 77, 103, 135, 136
acidity, 74, 116
acidosis, 74, 75, 77
acne, 129, 135
addicting, 98
addiction, 11, 41, 57, 98
addictive, 11, 12, 25, 27, 111
adenosine triphosphate, 71
ADHD, 1, 19, 112
age spots, 137
aging, 5, 14, 16, 48, 58, 59, 61, 65, 66, 68, 70, 71
alcohol, 25, 41, 42, 61, 75
alcoholic, 98
alkaline, 43, 44, 55, 60, 74, 75, 76, 77, 103, 106, 116
alkaline water, 44, 76,
alkalinity, 43, 44, 74, 76, 77, 106, 124
alkalosis, 76, 77, 107
Almond milk, 42
almonds, 12, 16, 32, 63, 79
aluminum, 45, 86

Alzheimer's disease, 45, 58, 61, 86, 137
AMA, 117, 126
American Medical Association, 117, 122, 124
amino acids, 35, 59, 64, 72, 136
anaerobic, 71, 116
aneurysms, 31
Antarctica, 101
antelope, 50
anti- inflammatory, 82
antibiotics, 35, 37 84, 127, 128, 135
antifungal, 107, 123
anti-inflammatory, 48, 121, 136
anti-oxidant, 33, 62, 66, 70, 72, 79, 80, 82, 83, 106, 113, 1121, 127, 135, 136, 137, 138
anti-pathogenic, 105, 112, 113, 114
antiseptic, 43, 128, 129, 137
antiviral, 82
apple cider vinegar, 76, 91, 134, 135, 136, 137
apples, 25, 61, 62, 90
apricot, 80, 83
arterial sclerosis, 20, 54, 61
arthritis, 58, 61, 68, 75, 82, 136, 138
artichokes, 91
aspartic acid, 72
aspirin, 137
Astaxanthin, 113
asthma, 39
ATP, 71

autism, 1, 19, 105, 113
avocado, 22, 32, 48, 90, 92

B

bacon, 24, 109
bacteria, 20, 42, 43, 54, 55, 57, 62, 63, 106, 116, 123, 125, 128, 129, 130, 134, 135, 138
bacterial, 57, 107, 117, 119, 123
baking soda, 106, 107, 123, 124
balance, 4, 9, 23, 39, 44, 48, 65, 67, 70, 81, 83, 103, 138
balsamic vinegar, 90
bananas, 80, 83
barbecuing, 86
barley, 54
basil, 80, 88
bay leaves, 89
beans, 22, 33, 63, 75, 88, 89
Beck Protocol, 125, 127, 130
beef, 25, 37, 57, 79, 80, 88, 90
beer, 42, 53
behavioral, 9, 20, 27, 112
Belarus, 102
bell pepper, 88, 90
berries, 48, 58, 61, 62, 90, 136
bicarbonate, 106
Big Business, 20
Big Medicine, 117, 118, 120, 122, 126, 130

Big Pharma, 54
bilberry, 82, 84
bile, 38, 118, 131, 133
birth defects, 87, 102
Black Cohosh, 82
bladder, 121
blood pressure, 10, 15, 28, 33, 38, 43, 81, 82, 106
blood purifier, 125, 126
Botulism, 57
Brazil nuts, 33, 62
bread, 21, 24, 25, 50, 51, 55, 56, 57, 75, 96
breakfast, 11, 20, 24, 48, 55, 56, 72, 85, 91, 92, 109, 113
breast, 32, 57, 116, 118
breastfed, 57
broccoli, 72, 80, 90, 92
bromelain, 62
Brussels sprouts, 80
Budwig Diet, 60
Budwig Protocol, 120
bullion, 89
burgers, 28, 93
butt, 9, 32, 33, 48, 65, 74, 92, 94
butter, 56, 91

C

cabbage, 53, 54, 83, 87, 89, 90
cactus, 48, 90, 92, 136
calcium, 20, 36, 38, 42, 54, 61, 63, 80, 104, 105
calorie, 5, 14, 15, 16, 22, 23, 24, 25, 28,

31, 33, 34, 39, 41, 48, 49, 50, 61, 62, 63, 72, 73, 88, 89, 90, 91, 92, 94, 95, 96
cancer, 1, 8, 19, 20, 33, 37, 42, 43, 45, 54, 55, 58, 60, 61, 62, 71, 73, 74, 76, 77, 80, 82, 83, 86, 100, 102, 104, 107, 112, 113, 115, 116, 117, 118, 119, 120, 121, 122, 123, 124, 125, 127, 128, 129, 132, 136, 138
Candida Albicans, 123
canola, 20, 22, 25
capitalistic, 53, 72, 110
carbohydrates, 21, 31, 32, 34, 48, 51
carbon, 60, 71, 73, 74, 75, 77, 86
carbon dioxide, 60, 73, 74, 75, 77
carbs, 20, 21, 22, 25, 26, 31, 32, 34, 48, 50, 51, 71, 72, 91
carcinogen, 86
cardio, 70, 71, 95
cardiovascular, 39, 83
Carl Zeiss, 116
carrots, 49, 72, 79, 83, 87, 89, 90, 91
cartilage, 4
cashews, 33, 90
Cast iron, 85
cauliflower, 90
cayenne, 58
celery, 49, 88, 89
Celiac, 26
cell rejuvenation, 14,

36, 39, 43, 59
Center for Disease Control, 116
ceramic, 44, 85, 86, 87
cereal, 20, 32, 55, 56
Cesium, 100, 104
Cesium-137, 100
chayote, 89
cheese, 25, 35, 39, 50, 57, 58, 71, 79, 80, 81, 82, 94, 96, 98
cheeseburgers, 75
chelating, 104, 105
chelation,104, 105, 106
chemo, 74, 83, 122
chemotherapy, 122
Chernobyl, 99, 100, 102
cherry, 103, 131, 132
chickens, 24, 37, 50, 51, 57, 79, 85, 88, 89, 109, 112, 116
chlorella, 105, 106
Chloride, 81
chlorine, 21, 128
chocolate, 103
cholesterol, 10, 15, 28, 35, 36, 38, 39, 40, 55, 62, 79, 83, 131, 136, 137, 138
chromium, 45, 82, 86, 105
cilantro, 105, 106
Cinnamon, 82
circulation, 82
circulatory, 22, 25, 33, 35, 36, 38, 54, 62, 105, 122
citrus, 61, 62, 136
coconut milk, 36
coconut oil, 22, 38, 39, 40, 48, 91, 131, 137, 138
colloidal silver, 122,
142

127, 128, 129
complex carb, 25
Congestive Heart
   Failure, 8
contamination, 100,
   101
cookware, 44, 45,
   85, 86
copper, 45, 82
corn, 20, 21, 22, 24,
   25, 37, 54, 56, 57,
   61, 89, 90
corn syrup, 24, 56
corruption, 53
cortisol, 49, 51, 72
cottonseed, 20, 22,
   25
cow, 24, 25, 42, 54,
   57, 66, 101, 109
Crabs, 36, 11
Cranberry, 83
crockpots, 87
Crohn's, 26
crustaceans, 113
cucumbers, 87, 90

D

dairy, 42, 54, 55, 57,
   58, 63, 64, 71,
   109, 118
dandelion, 53
Dandelion Root, 82
dandruff, 137
dark leafy greens, 80
debris, 14
deer, 59, 109
degenerative, 16, 45,
   67, 68
dementia, 58, 86
dermatitis, 137
detoxify, 27
diabetes, 15, 19, 20,
   25, 28, 41, 43, 58,
   62, 63, 73, 94, 95,
   97, 120, 121

diabetics, 62, 63,
   122, 136, 138
digestive, 20, 26, 34,
   35, 43, 49, 54, 55,
   56, 59, 60, 85, 95,
   123, 129, 133,
   134, 135, 138
Dimethyl Sulfoxide,
   121
dinner, 24, 25, 50,
   51, 87, 93, 95, 113
distilled water, 103,
   104
DMSO, 121, 122
DNA, 42, 65, 65, 105
Dr. Albert
   Schweitzer, 120
Dr. Bob Beck, 125
Dr. Johanna Budwig,
   58, 120
Dr. Max Gerson, 118,
   130
Dr. Otto Warburg,
   115
Dr. Royal Rife, 116
Dr. Tullio Simoncini,
   122
drug, 19, 28, 41, 121,
   126, 127
Dutch oven, 89, 90

E

earthquake, 100
Echinacea, 82
E-Coli, 37, 57
eczema, 58, 135, 137
EDTA, 105
egg, 15, 24, 35, 48,
   49, 57, 72, 81, 85,
   91, 92, 109
Elderberry, 82
electrolyte, 42, 80,
   81
electro-medicine,
   124, 125

Endo-skeletal, 4
Endoskeleton, 4
enzyme, 62, 81, 82
epidemic, 57, 67, 74
Epsom salts, 131,
   133, 134
erectile dysfunction,
   83
Eskimos, 32
estrogen, 60
Europe, 27, 43, 111,
   112, 119, 128
exercise, 2, 4, 10,
   13, 14, 15, 27, 41,
   49, 60, 65, 67, 68,
   69, 70, 71, 79, 80,
   94, 95, 97, 98

F

fat soluble, 38
fats, 2, 11, 16, 22,
   23, 24, 25, 31, 38,
   39, 40, 48, 57, 58,
   62, 91, 96, 131,
   133
FDA, 121
Ferdinand
   Sauerbruch, 119
fiber, 21, 22, 33, 34,
   62, 63
fibromyalgia, 105
fish, 32, 36, 37, 38,
   44, 66, 80, 81, 82,
   100, 102, 103
flax, 58
flaxseed, 22, 38
flaxseed oil, 22
flexibility, 4, 65, 70
fluoride, 21, 82, 124
Folate, 80
follicles, 135
fortified iron, 20, 54
France, 111
free radicals, 61, 62,
   70, 72

Free radicals, 61, 70
frequency generator,
   117, 118
fries, 11, 25, 34, 75,
   93, 94
fructose, 56, 57, 61,
   64, 90
fruit, 22, 33, 41, 48,
   60, 61, 62, 64, 72,
   73, 75, 81, 90, 92,
   109, 110, 113,
   134, 136
Fukushima, 100, 102
functionality, 70
fungus, 55, 123, 124,
   125, 135

G

gall bladder, 119,
   130, 131, 132
garden, 21, 28, 33,
   66, 109, 110
garlic, 25, 51, 87, 88,
   89, 90, 91
genes, 65, 66
genetic, 17, 27, 34,
   37, 81, 105, 112
Germany, 58, 112,
   116, 119, 120,
   128, 129
gingko biloba, 83, 84
Ginseng, 68
glands, 3, 67, 136
glass, 43, 44, 77, 86,
   109, 117, 128,
   133, 134
gluten, 26, 34
GMO, 20, 23, 24, 25,
   26, 27, 34, 35, 37,
   38, 43, 56, 57, 60,
   61, 62, 85, 113
goat, 42, 58, 113
grain, 21, 22, 24, 25,
   34, 39, 54, 55, 64,
   81, 82

grapefruit, 61, 131,
   133
Grapes, 83
Great Britain, 111
Greece, 111
Greenland, 101
gullible, 53, 103,
   113, 121, 122
gynecomastia, 42

H

H2O2, 128
H2O3, 128
hair, 26, 60, 80, 126,
   135
hamburger, 50
Hawaii, 107
HDL, 136
headaches, 83, 118,
   119
heart attack, 10, 15,
   35, 54, 55, 63

heart disease, 10, 15,
   41, 43, 54, 58, 63,
   73
heart rate, 36, 69,
   70, 73
heartburn, 135
heavy metals, 1, 45,
   104, 105, 106
height-weight
   proportion, 27, 31
herbal, 82, 84
heredity, 8, 36
Herxheimer, 14, 51,
   130
Herxheimer's
   Syndrome, 14
Hippocrates, 53
hips, 67
Hiroshima, 102
HIV, 125, 126
holistic, 19
Honey, 58, 83

hops, 42
hormone, 22, 32, 37,
   39, 41, 42, 49, 59,
   60, 69, 71, 72, 83,
   138
HPV, 116
hydrogen, 40, 128
hydrogen peroxide,
   128
hyperactivity, 20
hypertension, 15
hypothyroidism, 104

I

ice cream, 16, 51, 93
ignorant, 53, 103,
   113, 121
immune system, 63,
   69, 80, 81, 82, 84,
   123, 125, 126,
   130, 135, 138
impotence, 72
induction, 87
infections, 82, 84,
   138
insects, 37
insulin, 20, 41, 62,
   63, 122, 136, 138
insurance, 3, 66
intestines, 26, 34,
   106, 118, 131
intravenously, 127
iodine, 36, 81, 104
Ireland, 111
iron, 20, 55, 63, 81,
   82, 85, 89, 104,
   105
Italy, 111

J

jalapeno, 88, 89
Japan, 100, 102, 103,
   105
joint, 14, 38, 68, 75

juice, 40, 41, 76, 87, 89, 91, 110, 118, 131, 132, 133, 134

K

kale, 79, 80, 90
Kangen, 43
Kava, 83
kefir, 58
ketchup, 24
kidney, 5, 9, 10, 14, 23, 39, 41, 43, 51, 54, 61, 74, 83, 103, 106, 130, 138
knees, 67

L

Lactate, 71
lactic acid, 71
Laetrile, 80
lamb, 35, 38
lard, 38, 96
L-Arginine, 62, 63, 105
laziness, 2, 10, 28, 47, 67
LDL, 136
Leaky Gut Syndrome, 138
Lean meats, 64
legislation, 19, 53, 117
legume, 33, 63
legumes, 30, 53, 67, 68
lemon, 75, 76, 89, 90, 91, 133
lentils, 80
lettuce, 25, 50, 87, 90, 111
leukemia, 116
life expectancy, 60, 73, 99
life-changing, 68

ligaments, 4
lions, 59
Listeria, 57
liver, 14, 19, 31, 32, 35, 36, 38, 39, 41, 53, 54, 56, 72, 74, 80, 82, 83, 84, 118, 126, 130, 131, 132, 134, 136, 138
L-Methionine, 136
lobsters, 36
longevity, 13, 54, 57, 60, 64, 65, 70, 86
Los Angeles, 109, 112
lunch, 48, 50, 87
lungs, 3, 74, 76
lymphatic, 39, 115

M

macadamia nuts, 33
magnesium, 61, 63, 67, 104, 105
magnetic pulser, 126
magnetic pulses, 126
Malaysia, 137
male enlarged breasts, 42
male pattern baldness, 135
malic acid, 131, 132
malnourished, 5, 34
manganese, 105
Manganese, 82
Manhattan, New York, 119
margarine, 22, 24, 25, 40
Marijuana, 43
marinara, 11, 25, 50
marrow, 89
mayonnaise, 58, 91
media, 42, 53, 66, 103, 113, 118,

122, 123
medications, 15, 19, 61, 123, 125, 132, 137
memory, 83, 138
menopausal, 82, 83
mercury, 1, 36, 105, 113
metabolism, 5, 14, 15, 16, 32, 36, 38, 39, 49, 50, 59, 61, 63, 71, 95
microbe, 55, 63, 107, 124, 125, 127, 130, 136, 138
microbial, 71, 126
microbiologist, 116
microorganisms, 116, 117
Microwave, 86
milk, 20, 21, 24, 32, 35, 39, 42, 48, 51, 55, 57, 81, 109
Milk Thistle, 83
mineral, 20, 23, 33, 54, 61, 62, 79, 80, 81, 82, 84, 103, 104, 105
moisturizer, 137
molecules, 72
Molybdenum, 82
motivation, 9, 13, 15, 16, 17, 47
mozzarella, 96

muscle, 4, 5, 23, 31, 34, 35, 41, 49, 59, 65, 66, 67, 68, 69, 70, 71, 72, 75, 79, 80, 81, 83, 98
muscle soreness, 70
mushrooms, 80

N

Nagasaki, 102

NASA, 59
nausea, 14, 82
neurological, 85, 86
Niacin, 79
Nobel Prize, 62, 115, 116, 120
nopales, 48
nucleus, 63
nutrients, 4, 22, 23, 26, 28, 32, 33, 34, 35, 36, 37, 40, 42, 48, 49, 50, 51, 60, 62, 71, 72, 79, 84, 88, 91, 92, 97, 104, 105, 106, 132, 138
nutritionist, 75, 93, 94, 97, 98
nutritious, 15, 23, 26, 33, 40, 41, 49, 55, 63, 88, 89, 95, 96, 105
nuts, 22, 33, 34, 38, 48, 49, 51, 58, 62, 63, 64, 72, 75, 79, 80, 81, 82, 90

O

oats, 54
obesity, 19, 26, 27, 54, 56, 57, 67, 73, 74
olive oil, 22, 88, 90, 131
Omega 3, 36, 38, 39, 56
Omega 6, 38, 39, 56
onion, 25, 87, 88, 89, 90, 91, 92
Oranges, 80
oregano, 88, 89, 90, 91
organic, 21, 33, 38, 50, 58, 61, 62, 96, 112, 113, 118

organisms, 20, 36, 41, 43, 55, 59, 117, 125, 126, 127
organs, 3, 26, 31, 43, 54, 100, 126, 136
osteoarthritis, 104
osteoporosis, 4, 23, 43, 68, 104, 138
oxalate, 61
oxidative, 65
oxygen, 2, 8, 43, 44, 60, 70, 71, 73, 76, 77, 81, 116, 128, 129
ozonated water, 21, 43, 128, 129
ozone gas, 43, 128

P

Pacific Ocean, 100, 101, 102
pain-free, 68
Pancakes, 24
pancreas, 20, 26, 41, 138
Pantothenic Acid, 80
paparazzi, 123
papaya, 25, 62
parasites, 125, 130, 136
Paris, 111
Parkinson's disease, 58, 86
Pasadena, California, 117
pasteurization, 41, 109, 132
pastrami, 98

pathogens, 117, 124, 125, 126, 127, 129, 130, 136
pathologist, 116
peach, 80, 110
peanuts, 22, 33, 63,

110
Pears, 83
peas, 33
pepper, 24, 58, 88, 91
pepperoni, 96
pesticides, 21, 33, 61, 109, 129
petroleum, 44, 86, 112, 113
Peyton Rous, 116
pH, 43, 44, 60, 74, 75, 76, 77, 81, 124, 136
pharmaceutical, 19, 61, 115, 124, 126, 127
Philippines, 137
phosphorus, 63, 81
physical limitations, 7, 67, 68
physicist, 38, 125
phytonutrients, 105
pigs, 24, 37, 101, 109
Pine nuts, 90
pineapples, 62
pistachio, 80
pizza, 11, 16, 34, 50, 93, 94, 95, 96, 111
plastic, 27, 28, 44, 86
pleasure, 11, 28, 86, 93, 98, 110
plums, 25, 80
pneumonia, 127
poisonous, 21, 63
polio, 115
polio vaccines, 115
pollutants, 1, 19, 36
pollution, 1, 21, 36
pork, 37, 38, 57, 79, 88, 90, 109
Post Concussion Syndrome, 4
post workout, 71, 72
potassium, 63
potatoes, 12, 16, 21, 25, 61, 79, 83, 89,

90
Poultry, 37
power lifting, 67
pregnancy, 36, 105
prescription drugs, 26, 82, 132
pressed juices, 40
prime rib, 95
Probiotic, 43
propaganda, 23, 103, 113
prostate, 10, 33, 54
protein, 5, 10, 16, 20, 23, 24, 25, 32, 33, 34, 35, 36, 37, 38, 42, 48, 49, 50, 51, 54, 58, 59, 62, 63, 64, 71, 72, 80, 81, 88, 89, 91, 105, 106, 138
psoriasis, 58, 137

Q

quackery, 19, 117
quality of life, 2, 7, 8, 15, 28, 64, 65, 67, 68, 138

R

radiation, 74, 83, 86, 87, 99, 100, 101, 102, 103, 104, 105, 106, 113, 122, 123
radioactive, 100, 102, 103, 104
radishes, 90
ramen, 28
recovery, 16, 23, 35, 50, 51, 62, 69, 71, 72
red peppers, 80
regression, 66
repetitions, 68

replenish, 71, 72
reproductive, 26, 38, 54
restaurant, 23, 28, 50, 95, 111, 128
rheumatoid arthritis, 39, 42, 75, 76
Riboflavin, 79
rice, 21, 32, 50, 51, 54, 75
RNA, 105
Russia, 128, 129
rye, 54

S

safflower, 96
salad, 16, 24, 43, 50, 56, 76, 87, 90, 91,
salad dressing, 24, 43, 56, 90

salmon, 37, 113
salmonella, 37, 57
salt, 11, 24, 25, 26, 33, 63, 81, 88, 89, 91, 106, 110, 111, 112
San Diego, California, 120
sarcopenia, 66
Sausage, 96
scallion onions, 80
Seafood, 81
seals, 32
seaweed, 81
seeds, 34, 38, 58, 60, 62, 63, 64, 79, 80, 81, 82, 90
selenium, 33, 37, 62, 70, 82
sex, 11
sexual, 33, 43, 81
sheep, 35, 42, 58
shoulder, 67
silver, 126, 127, 128

skin, 3, 4, 14, 21, 31, 32, 33, 35, 80, 89, 119, 121, 129, 130, 135, 137
sleep, 14, 16, 50, 51, 59, 71, 83, 134
slow resistance interval training, 67, 68
smoking, 86, 98
snacks, 48, 49, 51, 113
Social Security, 58, 66
soda, 56, 106, 107, 123, 124
sodium, 33, 80, 81, 106, 124
sodium absorbate, 106
soft drinks, 20, 24
sour cherry juice, 131, 132
sour cream, 50
soy, 20, 25, 37, 42, 53, 59, 33
soybeans, 22, 43, 56, 59, 61, 63, 75, 85, 90
spaghetti, 11, 25, 50, 51, 88
Spain, 111
sperm, 42, 81
spinach, 48, 61, 80, 92
Spirulina, 87, 106
squash, 11, 50, 61, 88, 90
St. John's Wort, 83
stainless steel, 45, 86
staph infection, 129
sterility, 20, 86, 87
steroid, 54
stomach, 3, 22, 26, 44, 48, 57, 76, 81, 83, 92, 97, 98,

119, 126, 134, 135
stress, 15, 49, 65, 71, 83, 97, 132
stretching, 67
stroke, 10, 15, 35, 36, 41, 54, 55, 62, 122
Sublingual, 35
sugar, 11, 16, 20, 21, 22, 24, 25, 32, 41, 52, 51, 54, 55, 56, 61, 62, 63, 64, 71, 72, 73, 74, 76, 79, 82, 90, 110, 111, 112,132, 136, 138
sulfur, 58, 81
Sunflower seeds, 90
surgery, 74, 117, 130
sweet peppers, 90
synthetic, 40, 105, 113

T

tamales, 96
Teflon, 85, 86
tendencies, 1, 11, 98, 138
tendons, 4
testosterone, 42, 53, 72
Thiamin, 79
thighs, 31, 33, 48, 92
thyroid, 21, 33, 36, 42, 59, 60, 81, 86, 102, 104, 132
tigers, 59
Tijuana, Mexico, 120
Tokyo, 102
tomatoes, 21, 25, 48, 61, 62, 87, 88, 89, 90, 91, 92, 111, 112
topically, 127, 135, 137
tortilla, 24, 32, 55

toxins, 1, 13, 14, 19, 21, 31, 39, 51, 57, 59, 62, 86, 94, 104, 118, 130, 131, 132, 133, 136
trans fats, 25, 40
tsunami, 100
tuna, 100
turkey, 37, 79, 89
turmeric, 58, 83, 84, 89

U

Ukraine, 99, 102
United Nations, 106
United States, 37, 58, 72, 74, 100, 111, 112, 115, 119, 120, 121, 122, 128, 129
United States Olympic Team, 72
University of Southern California, 117
urinary tract, 83
urination, 33
urine, 9, 10, 14, 51, 100, 103, 113

V

varicose veins, 134, 135
vegetables, 22, 33, 34, 41, 48, 58, 59, 60, 61, 73, 75, 76, 79, 80, 81, 82, 87, 89, 90, 91, 92, 109, 110
vegetarian, 77, 132, 133, 134
veggies, 22, 49
Venison, 109
villi, 26, 34

vinegar, 21, 33, 61, 76, 77, 89, 90, 91, 106, 107, 134, 135, 136, 137, 138
viruses, 84, 116, 125, 127, 130
Vitamin A, 70, 79
Vitamin B1, 79
vitamin B12, 60, 80
Vitamin B17, 80
Vitamin B2, 79
Vitamin B3, 79
Vitamin B5, 80
Vitamin B6, 80, 83
Vitamin B9, 80
vitamin C, 80, 84, 105, 106, 124
vitamin D, 42, 60
Vitamin E, 56, 80
Vitamin K, 80
vitamins, 20, 23, 38, 54, 79, 80, 84, 122, 135
volunteers, 65

W

walnuts, 33, 90
water, 1, 3, 4, 10, 13, 19, 21, 24, 25, 26, 28, 31, 33, 35, 36, 41, 42, 43, 44, 54, 58, 60, 61, 62, 75, 76, 80, 82, 87, 89, 91, 100, 101, 102, 103, 104, 106, 122, 123, 127, 128, 129, 131, 133, 134
weight training, 66, 71
wheat, 25, 34, 54, 55, 96
Wheatgrass, 60
whey protein, 72
whipped cream, 103

148

white beans, 63
wine, 25, 88, 127
worms, 37
wrinkles, 137

Y

yeast, 24, 25, 55, 63,
82, 123, 134, 138
yoga, 4, 67, 70

Z

Zeolite, 104
zinc, 70, 81, 84, 105
zucchini, 25, 61, 91,
92

About The Author

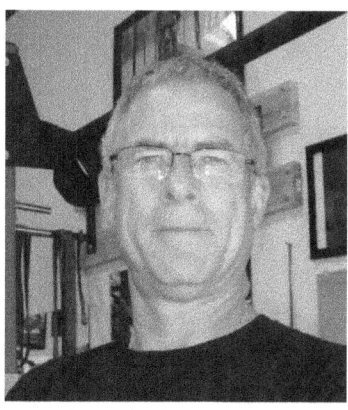

Michael Schlie is a former engineer who became tired of watching sick and overweight people struggle to survive throughout their days. Missing the engineering aspect of his life and tired of seeing humanity suffer, Michael decided to tackle the true interworkings of the human body. By treating his research as an engineering project, he discovered it was best to learn this information without the limitations brought on by formal education. Now certified as a personal trainer, weight loss expert and in sports nutrition, Michael wanted the world to learn from his personal journey. First and foremost, Michael prides himself on being a good father and loves to sing karaoke with his daughter. As much as he would love to be able to sing like Freddy Mercury or Steve Perry, he realizes everyone has their limitations.

For more information regarding cures and treatments found in Chapter 15, please go to **www.cancertutor.com**. Many of the diagrams and schematics regarding the Beck Protocol and other information regarding the use of DMSO can be found at the tremendous website.

www.ingramcontent.com/pod-product-compliance
Lightning Source LLC
Chambersburg PA
CBHW072122280526
45788CB00002B/512